Supporting Families & Carers

~

A Nursing Perspective

Supporting Families & Carers

~

A Nursing Perspective

Mary E. Braine

Senior Lecturer,
School of Nursing, Midwifery,
Social Work and Social Science,
University of Salford, UK

Julie Wray

Senior Lecturer/User and Carer Lead,
School of Nursing, Midwifery,
Social Work and Social Science,
University of Salford, UK

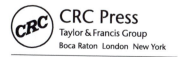

CRC Press
Taylor & Francis Group
Boca Raton London New York

CRC Press is an imprint of the
Taylor & Francis Group, an **informa** business

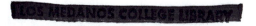

CRC Press
Taylor & Francis Group
6000 Broken Sound Parkway NW, Suite 300
Boca Raton, FL 33487-2742

© 2016 by Taylor & Francis Group, LLC
CRC Press is an imprint of Taylor & Francis Group, an Informa business

No claim to original U.S. Government works

Printed on acid-free paper
Version Date: 20160301

International Standard Book Number-13: 978-1-4987-0670-4 (Paperback)

Visit the Taylor & Francis Web site at
http://www.taylorandfrancis.com

and the CRC Press Web site at
http://www.crcpress.com

Contents

Foreword

I am delighted to write a few words to introduce *Supporting Families and Carers: A Nursing Perspective*. Julie Wray was a 2014–2015 Travel Scholar of the Florence Nightingale Foundation, and in the study she undertook for her scholarship, she looked at what helps to enhance family carers' experiences of healthcare. Her study and this book are highly topical and pertinent. Most people are likely to have caring responsibilities at some stage in their lives. With a rising population of older people and enhanced medical and technological capabilities, many of us will live longer with a variety of long-term conditions requiring help and support from families, friends and/or nursing and social care. Therefore, increasingly many of us will have the experience of caring not just for young members of our families but also for frail, elderly loved ones.

As a nurse, I myself have had the personal experience of caring for a loved one: when I took a sabbatical to nurse my mother at home in the final two months of her terminal illness. Whilst this was one of the great privileges of my life to be trusted and have the capability to meet the final needs of a loved one in her preferred place of death, I know how important it is to have support in order to maintain one's own resilience and meet the challenges with compassion and equanimity.

Carers are central to contemporary health services, and working with carers is fundamental to the delivery of high-quality person- and family-centred nursing care. Being a carer has a significant impact on people's lives, and awareness of carers' needs is increasing in the healthcare professions. How to work effectively in partnership with patients and users, but also their carers, has a growing evidence base which nurses need to access to inform their practice. In this book, Julie and Mary Braine harness their wealth of direct personal experience, their in-depth knowledge of clinical practice and their expertise in supporting student nurses across diverse areas of care to synthesise the growing literature in this area and offer practical interventions to support this key group of patients/users and carers.

The Florence Nightingale Foundation, as the living legacy of Florence Nightingale, awards scholarships to nurses and midwives which support research and scholarly activity in the crucial areas of care that truly make a difference to the experience of patients and their carers.

Professor Elizabeth Robb, OBE
Chief Executive of the Florence Nightingale Foundation
London, United Kingdom

Acknowledgements

We thank the staff at CRC Press for their support. Help from Stephanie Enright, Jean Parnell, Sophie Dishman, Helen Hills, Paul Moran, Robert Finnigan and Sue Bellass is acknowledged. We also thank Salford Carers Centre for their support and insights. Finally, and perhaps most importantly, we thank the University of Salford user and carer groups, the many student nurses who have inspired us over the years with their experiences and stories and the many families and carers we have met during the course of our nursing careers.

Introduction

The caregiving experience is unique to each family and caregiver, and this experience is often likened to that of a 'roller coaster ride' with many ups and downs reliant upon their loved ones' individual illnesses or disease trajectories. Thus, caring for a relative or close friend is not a static process as their needs change when their condition alters. Moreover, this caregiving experience does not occur in a vacuum but rather is influenced by a number of complex psychosocial factors which all impact the coping skills of the carer. The art of nursing is critical in developing therapeutic relationships and to understanding these experiences. This book aims to offer insights into the fundamental principles of caring for families and carers irrespective of age, gender, ethnicity, sexuality or religion. Our aim in writing this book is to facilitate nurses to understand and support family caregivers in their carer roles. The book is intended to provide a unique resource to inform nursing practice and learning at all levels.

We have sought to pull together examples from our own research, personal experiences, clinical practice (MEB in acute care and JW in community) alongside key theories and our years of experience teaching nursing students. Our own values and beliefs formed since we started our nursing careers many years ago remain strong in that we believe the goal of nursing is to assist family members in maintaining and optimising levels of wellness and to enhance their health and well-being. Our belief is that we can't understand the patient without understanding the family and the patient's role within the family. We also take the broad view that caregiving that involves providing care for a dependent family member has real potential to enhance recovery and well-being of patients and family members. Creating empowering relationships between patients, carers and nurses has the capacity to make a genuine difference in people's lives. In support, we hope that you, the reader, will also revisit your own beliefs and values with respect to supporting families and caregivers.

Current demographical trends have impacts such as longer life expectancy, rising older population, co-production, shared decision-making and increasing trend towards community care. With advancements in technological knowledge and medical capabilities, more families engage in day-to-day care to more complex care tasks. Of course, this may be in the short term, as in post-discharge day care or short illness, but for many this means providing both long-term practical and emotional support. Given the rising expectations that carers will be undertaking much more care in the future, there is an imperative to include families and carers as key partners and collaborators. Of course, for many families and carers, their caring responsibility can be all consuming; furthermore, we cannot assume that the caring role has been chosen. It can just happen. The nature of illness and disease is that a care role occurs unexpectedly and suddenly, resulting in immersion into the world of providing care to a now-dependent loved one without any preparation. Thus, we cannot make assumptions about carers and families in terms of their ability to cope and manage their role, as carers are not a homogenous group; they are as different as all people in the population. Whilst we recognise that caregivers' experiences are not linear in nature but rather are a complex cocktail of experiences, we aim to disentangle the complexity of family and carers experiences.

Understanding the perspective of carers is an essential aspect of nursing, and we offer detailed information and theories to enable insights and knowledge acquisition. That said, our book is not meant to be historical but it is our effort to contextualise some of the pertinent issues such as terms used, guiding principles and underpinning theories. The terms 'carer' and 'caregiver' are used interchangeably throughout the book to refer to the person who provides care to another person who is dependent on him/her for help.

We feel that whilst theories may be removed from the real world of nursing, all nursing practice is underpinned and guided by various theories. We believe that theories and concepts (the building blocks of theory) play an important role in helping us to both understand the actions and behaviours of others and provide theoretical rationales to guide specific nursing actions. Also, in order to grasp and understand the concepts and theories that underpin our understanding of the behaviours and feelings that families and caregivers may experience, we believe it is important to examine the origins of these concepts and theories. For this reason, some past contextual backgrounds to these theories and concepts are offered although this is not meant to be all encompassing.

The book is divided into seven chapters; in Chapters 1 and 2, we set the scene for contextualising care, and Chapters 3 through 5 provide theoretical frames to understanding the caregiving experiences. Whilst we have presented theories and concepts in Chapters 3 through 5 as separate entities in the real world of people's lives, these concepts merge together within the whole experience of 'being and doing' caregiving within a person's unique context. Finally, Chapters 6 and 7 provide practical perspectives for nursing. We start in Chapter 1 by exploring how the informal carer role has evolved over time, covering terms and some statistics before discussing tasks in detail. In Chapter 2, we shed light on the concept of family, the most enduring institution in the world, followed by a discussion regarding function of the family and family dynamics along with an overview of grand family theories. There is no doubt that families are complex, and in order to understand the patient's role and position within the family and the interaction between the two, we feel it is worth drawing upon theoretical perspectives that have stood the test of time.

Stress and coping theories dominate the thinking about the outcomes of caregiving. In Chapters 3 and 4, we explore some of these various theoretical models of caregiving that help to explain the relationships among caregiver stress, psychosocial resources and caregiver well-being and how caregivers adjust and adapt to their role. Chapter 3 examines the stress process, stressors and theoretical understandings of stress and how this relates to caregiving. Adjusting and adapting to the role of carer is a challenge and so Chapter 4 delves into the roots of the caregiving mediators of stress. This chapter also looks at the actions and perceptions of the family caregiver and resources available to them that may help to alter stressful situations that they are faced with as they attempt to cope.

In deciding to write this book, an incentive was to pull together the increasing body of literature concerning the effects of caregiving and associated demands on the health and well-being of families and carers. Whilst the literature tends to be dominated by the negative experience with deleterious effects on physical and emotional health and well-being, we aim to provide in Chapter 5 a more rounded view. Caregiving is not a uniformly negative experience but one that can have both positive and negative consequences for health and well-being. For many carers, there is a juggling of their own needs with the needs of their loved ones; and for some, there is coping, acceptance and making the best of being in their caregiving role; whilst for others, there is positive growth. This chapter will explore the literature that points to the caregiver's negative experiences of caregiving, but also the positive effects of caregiving albeit a relatively small and emerging body of literature.

Nurses may need to intervene in order to help supporting families and carers achieve their goals and prevent ill health. Chapter 6 aims to provide an overview of some key interventions that focus on providing family-focused care that assists families and caregivers to function. Interventions include training and education programs, problem-solving skills, information technology–based support and formal approaches to planning care which take into account the specific needs of carers.

The notion of enabling the family to be involved in care, particularly in an institutional setting such as a hospital which can both be controlling and creating barriers for partnership working, is explored in Chapter 7. It is in this chapter that we explore some of the lost opportunities and obstacles to supporting families and carers and how connecting with the family may be enhanced. We have included some commentary from carers and people who work with carers to highlight salient points, with a desire to encourage you to think and reflect on what you might do in certain situations. There is no doubt that nurses are in privileged positions; how they act and interact matters in the lives of patients and their carers. Where empowering collaborations form through triad partnerships, there is an opportunistic window to work with families and carers.

Context of the Carer

Introduction

This chapter begins by providing a brief historical context alongside a section on definitions of carers, followed by an overview of a range of terms used in the literature and types of care typically undertaken. What is important to note is that the term 'carer' is used extensively in the United Kingdom (and in countries such as the United States, Canada and Australia) in health and social care policy (Molyneaux et al. 2011) and yet the term 'family' or 'relative' tends to be the preferred one in other European countries. Regardless of the preference of terms, what needs to be acknowledged is how important the role is economically, as billions of pounds are saved that would otherwise have to be spent on health and social care services. This chapter also covers several highlights from the UK census data in regard to numbers of carers with reference to ethnicity, age and hours dedicated to caregiving. Then, a discussion on carer awareness, caregiving tasks and responsibilities follows.

Growing interest in carers and carer awareness is becoming a priority in the United Kingdom. We have noted that over the past 20 years, there has been an explosion of interest and research into caring, 'family carer' and carers. With the availability of the UK census data (ONS 2001, 2011), we now have a better understanding of the prevalence, impact and experiences of carers. Of course, there is more to learn and know about in terms of their relationships with services and professionals, notably nurses. The ways in which carers are valued and involved as partners in care can vary considerably. For example, being able to understand and negotiate caring between the professional and carer, particularly in the hospital setting, is a real challenge (Allen 2000). By starting this book with a chapter on the context of carers, we seek to set the scene by offering a deeper understanding of carers before exploring the family, which follows in Chapter 2, so as to inform your understanding and knowledge base. Typically, people do not expect or plan to be carers – 'it just happens', and it can happen suddenly or gradually. There is temporal nature to being a carer or caregiver in that the role and experience is sequential and one can move in and out of caring. In addition, with the trend of 'carer of carers', which is the movement between the two roles of being a patient and carer (Marriott 2013), we need to be mindful of the dynamic nature of informal 'unpaid' caregiving. Caring can become a way of life but knowing of the carers' existence and respecting them is important as their 'job' (role) can be long, lonely and hard with limited support. Although it needs to be stated that in the United Kingdom from April 2015, the Care Act 2014 and the Children and Families Act 2014 ambitiously seek to change this stance by improving the rights and recognition of carers.

Fundamentally, the nature of human beings is that we *reach out* to help others (e.g. family and loved ones), sometimes known as the 'ethical demand' or 'ethical care' (Agard and Maindl 2009). In relation to nursing, Benner et al. (1999) have described these phenomena as 'human pull'; that said, we recognise that when carers and nurses come together, different reaching out factors and incentives come into play. Being able to understand one another requires knowledge, skills and moral incentives to work together; moreover, we suggest a set of values and beliefs that embrace caregiver and family involvement. Before exploring these attributes in more detail, a brief overview is offered in relation to origins of the word 'carer'.

Historical Background

Allen (2000) points out that following the 1959 Mental Health Act, a change in the division of labour between formal and informal carers emerged in the United Kingdom with the idea of community care. At the outset, community care had an emphasis towards care *in* the community, but in the 1970s, this shifted to mean care *by* the community, and Finch (1990) noted this subtle shift as a distinct policy feature of the time. Clearly, this shift placed reliance upon good citizenship, in other words *informal* caring (presumably *willingness*) that would be largely unpaid and voluntary. Interestingly, it was in the late 1970s that the term 'carer' started to appear in the literature; up until this time, carers were for the most part invisible and featured little in policy and research activities (Conn 2006). Typically, there was an expectation that carer roles were an integral part of family life as such; being a carer was informal and a private matter, certainly not a public one. For decades, family carers were unseen within society and it was during the UK government public policies on *care in the community* that public knowledge of the existence of *informal* carers began to emerge. 'Caring' and 'carers' were rather generic and entwined terms during this period, and Conn (2006, p. 6) highlights that

> The real strength of the generic term 'carer' lay in it being utilised by the emerging carers lobby, [what is currently known as Carers UK], who began to bring pressure to bear on government to recognise carers as a distinct group within our population [UK] with commonality of need and to acknowledge them in the rhetoric and reality of social policy.

As a consequence, the term has become well accepted in everyday discourse, health and social care policy, literature and research and has gained national recognition in the United Kingdom. Indeed the Nursing and Midwifery Council (NMC) in the United Kingdom has included support for carers in its publications and guidance as an essential requirement for all registrants and students for over a decade. Notably, carer identification and support and assistance for carers became a high priority for district and community nursing in 2001 (NMC 2001). At the same time within nurse education, inclusion and consideration of carers manifested in curricula within the *service user* and public involvement discourses and expectations of family-centred theories and principles. Perhaps broader terms have evolved, but within nursing ideology, the importance of family and friends in the care of significant others was explicitly documented by nursing theorists over 50 years ago, for example, Patricia Benner, Virginia Henderson, Dorethea Orem and Jean Watson.

Case Study

Consider this comment from a nurse:

> When I trained as a nurse in the 1980s I don't recall the term carer being used; we were taught to consider and include relatives and families. I knew that relatives and families would take over caregiving when patients went home but we didn't call them carers.

– Anonymous nurse comment

You may resonate with this comment or have met nurses who have said similar, so it is worth thinking about what impact the growth of the term 'carer' has on nursing and nurses in their everyday practice. (Make some notes.)

Interestingly, it is worth mentioning at this juncture that Molyneaux et al. (2011) critique the term 'carer' for its passive nature and undervalued connotations in how it is used politically and in the context of UK health and social care polices. The argument here is that the term 'carer' is ineffective in recognising the relationship between carers and those being cared, as, for the most part, it infers burden and fails to capture the possibility of reciprocal relationships and access to appropriate support. Heron (1998) draws a distinction between the political meaning (carers as a group who require a policy response) and the personal meaning (provides an identity and a role/membership of a group of people with similar concerns). Molyneaux et al. (2011) suggest that the term 'carer' is a label, and, as such, is disempowering and hostile with the scope to divide people creating discrimination and a rift for those in receipt of care who can be left vulnerable. They favour a universal adoption of a relationship-based description of caring, in that the term 'carer' is clarified on an individual basis according to the relationship to the care recipient, for example, terms such as family, dependent and, in the long term, 'care assistant'. Paradoxically, as a measure of the value and importance that carers save the UK economy, there was a campaign in the United Kingdom to give the word 'carer' protected status (Lloyd 2006), whereby its use would be confined to describing the activity of the many 'informal care' as opposed to health and social services supplied by paid workers. We will return to this discussion later in this chapter but for now we move onto to discuss some widely used definitions of carers.

Definitions of Carers

According to the Carers Trust, a dedicated UK charity that offers help and support and leads on taking action and provides advice for unpaid carers, 'carer' is defined as follows:

> Anyone who cares, unpaid, for a friend or family member who due to illness, disability, a mental health problem or an addiction cannot cope without their support.

– Carers Trust (2014)

This definition is well accepted and is cited in UK national policy, literature and materials pertaining to health and social care (e.g. DH 2008a,b). Although other terms such as 'family caregiver' and 'informal caregiver' are used, they essentially mean the same thing as they all refer to an unpaid family member, friend or neighbour who provides care to an individual who has an acute or chronic condition and needs assistance to perform a variety of tasks, from personal care to assistance with taking medications to tube feeding (Reinhard et al. 2008). The level of care and assistance varies considerably. Informal care does not involve payment or government regulation, as distinct from formal care that is paid and/or regulated.

An 'informal' carer can be of any age; this includes children, young people and adults, without whose help their family member, partner or friend would not be able to manage alone.

It is important to say that carers are not a homogeneous group in society but they are as different as the population at large, and each situation is unique. The common feature is that they care for someone who needs help and assistance and that becoming a carer can occur to anyone at any time regardless of status. Furthermore, it has been noted by White (2013) that carers are a socially and demographically diverse group, and as the demand for care is projected to grow*, it is increasingly likely for people to become providers of care at some point in their lives. Of course this can be within a family context, as friend or neighbour, the point being caregiving is highly likely to affect everyone in UK society over time (DH 2013a,b).

Typically in most societies today with ageing population and demographic changes, there has been an emergence of what is termed 'the sandwich generation' – those people sandwiched between ageing parents who need care and/or help and their own children. Such people can find themselves becoming a 'sandwich carer' providing simultaneous care to their young or adolescent children and at the same time becoming a carer to an older family member or friend (Chisholm 1989). Sandwich generation caregivers are typically aged 45–60 years who simultaneously care for a dependent young child and ageing parents.

Thinking Box

Do you know of someone like this? Perhaps you have met them in practice or in your personal life; did you recognise their dual roles as sandwich carers?

Were you aware of any issues that they faced? If not, can you imagine any issues they may face?

Other Terms

Over the years, with more knowledge and insights into the world of carers, distinct features have emerged about the nature of caring roles. To understand these features, other terms have evolved, which are outlined in Table 1.1. On the one hand, the terms can blur, and absolute boundaries between the different terms may well be not so clear in practice and people's lives. However, they are offered here by way of insight into what they mean.

Of note is a less familiar term, 'advocate' carer, which refers to a family member or caregiver who undertakes minimal direct caregiving tasks but acts as an 'advocate' for a loved one, family member or patient. This can be from any distance and can include indirect tasks as outlined in the "Caregiving Tasks/Responsibilities" section, but, in addition, this type of carer plays a strong advocacy role on behalf of the care recipient. In other words, this carer 'stands up for others' and is a strong voice for those who are less able to speak up or articulate their own needs.

As shown in Table 1.1, caregivers have been described as 'hidden patients' (Fengler and Goodrich 1979), 'secondary patients' (Reinhard et al. 2008) and, more recently, as the 'extended arm of the health professional' (Norlyk and Martinsen 2013). What a

---

* Due to international ageing population trends (see UN 2013; WHO 2014) and medical advances in treatments for genetic disorders, critical care, cancers and long-term conditions.

Table 1.1 Examples of other terms used for carers as seen in the literature

Term	Meaning
Career carer	Likening caring to a career with carer's experiencing transitions, key events and roles change over time same as a career. Montgomery and Kosloski (2000) suggest: 'caring is like a career with a "beginning discernable temporal direction and end"'. Career carers often see themselves as experts too. A distinction here is the movement into the post-caring phase (when a loved one dies).
Compound carer	Compound caregivers are those parents who are already providing considerable caregiving responsibilities for their son/daughter who subsequently becomes a caregiver for an additional family member (Perkins and Haley 2010).
Distance carer	People who provide any kind of meaningful support to a relative but do so from a distance (Carers UK 2011).
Expert carer	Carers who are established in that they have been caring for a family member or significant other (e.g. friend or neighbour) for some time. Typically, there is a level of dependency and an established caregiving relationship with a relative or loved one.
Grandparent carer	An emerging group of carers includes grandparents raising their own grandchildren, i.e., their own children's children, often due to relationship breakdown, violence or illness. An estimated 200,000 grandparents provide full-time care in the United Kingdom, and this figure is rising.
Hidden patients	Carers who are not recognised as a carer will go unseen, unrecognised and hidden from professionals. Though not always, such carers can be children, young people and women (Fengler and Goodrich 1979).
Placement carer	Carers who place a family member into a long-term care setting, where the role changes for that caregiver, whereby new relationships and interactions must be negotiated with staff, residents and families of other residents. The caregiver must relinquish her role as the primary provider of care recipient's personal care. Limited hands-on care evolves, but placement carers may find that there are new roles to be fulfilled.
Primary carer	Primary carer is the family member deemed to bear the most responsibility in caring for the injured (mainly mothers and wives) (Perlesz et al. 2000).
Sandwich carer	These carers provide simultaneous care to their young or adolescent children and at the same time act as carers to an older family member or friend.
Secondary carer	Secondary carers are those who are considered to be next in line to take on most responsibility (mostly fathers and eldest siblings) (Perlesz et al. 2000).

(Continued)

Table 1.1 (*Continued*) Examples of other terms used for carers as seen in the literature

Term	Meaning
Secondary patients	Carers could be recognised but their needs and concerns can be perceived to be less important than the patients; they are viewed as secondary or are ignored (Reinard et al. 2008).
Serial carers	Serial carers engage in cyclical caring and post-caring primarily due to a sense of family obligation.
Tertiary carer	Tertiary carers follow on from secondary carers in taking on the next most responsibility (mainly siblings) (Perlesz et al. 2000).
Young carer	Young carers include children and young people under 18 years old (aged 5–17) who provided unpaid care for family members, friends, neighbours or others because of long-term physical or mental ill health, disability or problems relating to old age.

Note: This is not an exhaustive list.

family caregiver and an informal caregiver have in common is that they are 'carers' with knowledge and expertise of the care recipient/family member. That said, it was way back in 1979 that Fengler and Goodrich (1979) found that carers are often referred to as 'hidden patients' as their psychological, physical and emotional stresses may go unnoticed due to the primary focus being on the needs of the care recipient. In 1954, Reverend Mary Webster at the age of 31 gave up her work to become a carer for her elderly parents. Feeling isolated in her caring role and thinking that others may be in a similar predicament, she turned to the newspapers. Bringing this private issue into the public domain saw the launch of the carer's movement, and the charity Carers UK was established in 1965 (Carers UK 2011). In the United Kingdom, there are numerous other charities that seek to support carers – Carers Trust (formerly the Princess Royal Trust), Care for Carers (careforcares. org.uk), Alzheimer's Association, Parkinson's UK, MIND and Rethink Mental Illness, to mention just a few.

We will return to definitions and roles that carers take on in relation to working with families and carers in Chapter 7. At this stage, what we seek to convey is the dynamic nature and complexity of assigning terms to caring in relation to usage in everyday discourse, UK policy documents and the literature. Regardless of the words, it is worth briefly considering that in terms of identity, caregivers can see themselves as having multiple identities and roles. As a role becomes aligned to one's sense of self, the individual, in this context carer, tends to behave in accordance with the identity of that role, i.e., 'carer'. By doing this, one can verify themselves in order to secure acknowledgement and visibility. Carer identity is influenced by the personal constructs of identity and social meanings of identity, both of which influence the positions that carers as a community and as an individual are seen in society at large.

Low Status

Accepting the term 'carer' can be challenging for people who see what they are doing is simply caring for a loved one, a family member, neighbour or friend, either temporarily or for long term (Hughes et al. 2013). It can be regarded as an expectation, obligation or duty and a basic function of family and community life (Montogmery 1999). Carers UK and the Princess Royal Trust (largest UK carer charities) dedicate much of their efforts to not only raising awareness to the plight of carers but also unpacking the label carer.

The term 'carer' has connotations with low status and can be disconnected from family relationships or loved ones, and it can be viewed as a label that people don't like, as highlighted by the following comments:

> I found it, the word carer really strange as I am his wife and I am caring for him, that's what I am doing being a wife, what's this carer word? I love him, I care for him, is that a carer?...

> —A carer (p/c 2013)

> My mother was a carer, she looked after dad who had multiple sclerosis for 15 years till he died. Of course in those days there was no such thing as being a carer, she just saw herself as his wife

> —A carer (Heron 1998)

The dimension of low status in part could be aligned to perceptions people have of the nature of caring duties and the language used in the context of carers. For example, having to undertake personal care such as washing, feeding, dressing and toileting can feel low in status. Losing control over one's own life and dealing with increasing levels of dependency and uncertainty can add to the perception of low status. Informal caring can be all-consuming. Carers often speak about their loss of identity and how they grapple with facing an uncertain future identity that can bring increased isolation and social, emotional and financial burden (Allen 2000; Cronin et al. 2014). Hugh Marriot in his book *Selfish Pig* (2013) states, 'we didn't apply for this job; most of us don't have a vocation for it; we are certain we are not much good at it and we have had no training' (p. 9). As a long-term carer for his wife, Marriot brings into the open issues that arise 'behind closed doors' in the lives of the many carers – the realities, he says, are often not addressed, and 'officials' too often fail to understand the workload and complexities facing carers day in and day out. His view is that too often the role is dismissed and devalued by friends and officials (health and social care professionals).

Aligned to low status, there can even be a reluctance to accept the word 'carer' due to feelings of stigma and perceived negative attitudes of the word. Stigma can be a real issue for young carers, in particular amongst their peers and at school. Whether real or perceived, children and young people who find themselves as carers face unique challenges that are different from those experienced by adult carers.

This sense of negative attitude can apply to anyone who finds themselves in the role of caring. Of course, the ways in which people adjust to the word and all that it infers to them and their situation are highly individual, but there is no getting away from the possibilities that one can feel under scrutiny from the external world. Often the word 'carer' is associated with a service that provides personal care, and in this context it is paid care or 'hired help'. For the purpose of our book, we focus entirely upon unpaid carers. That said, in practice, the perceptions can be very different for different people.

The visibility and experiences of young carers are even more complex and notably hidden, ignored or invisible. Efforts to raise not just awareness of young carers existence but the impact caring has upon their lives has been a feature of many charities and UK public policy. For example, in 2013, the UK Children's Society (Hounsell 2013) published an important study on the differential impact that caring has on young carers compared to children who are not carers. As might be expected, their education, employment and life chance opportunities are affected significantly, and, as a group, young carers face disadvantages that stay with them into later life. Strengthening young carers' rights and seeking to provide better outcomes are features of current policy (Hounsell 2013), but ensuring that young carers are identified, offered tailored support and are not hidden remains a challenge. In the North West region of England, a beacon carers' centre in Salford has sought to raise awareness of young carers through commissioned films.

Watch this film: *We're Not Different, We Just Do Different Things* (2012); https://www.youtube.com/watch?v=aHO8iRSuxyc.

Thinking Box

Make a note of what you consider to be the issues raised here.

How might this family be helped?

Who could have helped them?

Do you think stigma was an issue for the children?

How could this be handled?

In the context of this film, opportunities were lost, whereby benefits for, and with, the family as a unit could have occurred. Of course, the information revealed on the health status of the mother in this film is minimal; regardless, we are exposed to the plight of the children in seeking to cope with and manage their situation. Clearly, recognising or identifying carers is everyone's responsibility. In Chapters 6 and 7, we present detailed information on the types of support, interventions and services available to families and carers.

Moving on to some numbers now by way of illustration to further contextualise carers, we provide only a brief overview here (more details can be obtained from the UK census data at the ONS website, www.ons.gov.uk).

Numbers

The UK 2011 census found that the proportion of unpaid carers and the amount of care provided varied greatly amongst ethnic groups (Table 1.2). It can be seen in Table 1.2 that British (11.1%), Irish (11.0%) and Gypsy or Irish traveller (10.7%) were amongst the highest providers of unpaid care in England and Wales. Also White and Black African (4.9%), Chinese (5.3%), White and Asian (5.3%) and other White (5.3%) ethnic groups were amongst the lowest providers of unpaid care.

Carers are vital to the well-being and independence of thousands of people and the number of carers is constantly increasing. For example, in the 2011 census survey, it was estimated that there were around 6 million carers in England and Wales (ONS 2013; http://www.ons.gov.uk/ons/guide-method/census/2011/carers-week/index.html) compared to 5.2 million in 2001. What this tells us is that approximately 1 in 10 of the UK population is an unpaid carer supporting a friend or family member. More specifically, in England there were 5.41 million unpaid carers and 0.37 million in Wales, which equates to between 7% and 14% of the total population across England and Wales (White 2013). Given these figures, there is no doubt that nurses and other health professionals will come into contact with many carers during their professional practice, although not

Table 1.2 Ranked proportions of total unpaid care provision and the extent of unpaid care provided by the ethnic group, England and Wales, 2011

	1–19 hours of unpaid care	20–49 hours of unpaid care	50 or more hours of unpaid care	Total unpaid care (1–50+ hours)
White: English/Welsh/Scottish/ Northern Irish/British	7.1	1.4	2.6	11.1
White: Irish	6.7	1.4	2.9	11.0
White: Gypsy or Irish Traveller	4.4	1.9	4.4	10.7
Black/African/Caribbean/Black British: Caribbean	6.4	1.5	1.9	9.8
Asian/Asian British: Indian	5.9	2.0	1.9	9.7
Asian/Asian British: Pakistani	4.8	1.9	2.4	9.1
Asian/Asian British: Bangladeshi	4.7	1.8	2.3	8.8
Other ethnic group: Any other ethnic group	4.4	1.5	1.8	7.7
Asian/Asian British: Other Asian	3.9	1.5	1.5	6.9
Black/African/Caribbean/Black British: Other Black	4.2	1.2	1.4	6.9
Mixed/multiple ethnic group: White and Black Caribbean	3.8	1.0	1.2	6.1
Mixed/multiple ethnic group: Other mixed	4.0	0.9	1.1	6.0
Other ethnic group: Arab	3.0	1.3	1.8	6.0
Black/African/Caribbean/Black British: African	3.1	1.3	1.2	5.6
White: Other White	3.2	0.9	1.2	5.3
Mixed/multiple ethnic group: White and Asian	3.6	0.8	0.9	5.3
Asian/Asian British: Chinese	3.4	0.8	1.0	5.3
Mixed/multiple ethnic group: White and Black African	3.1	0.8	0.9	4.9

Source: Census – Office for National Statistics.

all will identify themselves as a carer. It is also the case that many adult and young carers remain hidden and often unsupported in taking on levels of care (Laing and Sprung 2013). Nurses can play an important role in providing support to carers. Although UK government policy places emphasis on integrated approaches to identifying, involving and supporting carers (DH 2010a, 2012, 2013a,b), every health professional has a responsibility and role to play.

Significant context factors such as the rapidly ageing world population are important to be aware of in the landscape of carers. Of note, the World Health Organisation (WHO) has stated as follows:

> Between 2000 and 2050, the proportion of the world's population over 60 years will double from about 11% to 22%. The absolute number of people aged 60 years and over is expected to increase from 605 million to 2 billion over the same period.
>
> – WHO (2014)

Longer life expectancies and ageing baby boomers will also increase the number (UN 2013; WHO 2014) and percentage of people living with long-term conditions, in particular neurodegenerative diseases such as Alzheimer's disease. In relation to disease trends, we know that in Europe approximately 10 million people suffer from dementia, with a worldwide estimation of 35 million people (Alzheimer's Disease International 2009). It is expected that these numbers will rise considerably to around 14 million by 2030 and 19 million by 2050. The trends are mirrored in the case of all neurodegenerative diseases throughout the Western world. For example, in the United Kingdom alone, approximately 1 in 500 people (approximately 127,000) has Parkinson's disease (Parkinson's UK 2013), which is the second most prevalent degenerative neurological condition in the country.

Young Carers

In 2011, there were 177,918 young unpaid carers (5–17 years old) in England and Wales. Of these, 54% were girls and 46% were boys. Within England, the North West had the highest proportion of young carers providing unpaid care at 2.3%, whereas the South East had the lowest proportion at 1.9% (Table 1.3). Overall, Wales had the highest proportion of young carers providing unpaid care at 2.6% (Table 1.3).

An increase in the number of unpaid carers aged 5–17 was observed in all regions between 2001 and 2011 (Table 1.3). In England and Wales combined, the number of young unpaid carers increased by almost 19% during this period. The South East had the largest increase of 41.2%, which equates to an additional 7282 young unpaid carers, whilst the smallest increase was seen in the North East at just 1.7%, an additional 135 young unpaid carers.

Young carers are members of families both immediate and extended and are often the sole or primary carer within the immediate family unit, yet they are possibly the ones who are most invisible to professional agencies (including health professionals). If we look at each caring situation as a family unit, in which all members may have caring roles, we stand the chance of acknowledging more young people as carers. This whole-family approach will also support the physical and mental well-being of the young carer themselves, reducing the need for long-term intervention and specialist support and enabling them to have the same life opportunities as their 'non-carer peers'.

Table 1.3 Proportion, numbers and percentage increases of unpaid carers aged 5–17 years between 2001 and 2011 in England and Wales

Country/region	Proportion providing unpaid care		Number of young unpaid carers		Percentage increase between 2001 and 2011
	2001 (%)	2011 (%)	2001	2011	
England and Wales	1.7	2.1	149,929	177,918	18.7
England	1.7	2.1	139,188	166,363	19.5
Wales	2.2	2.6	10,741	11,555	7.6
North East	1.8	2.1	7,808	7,943	1.7
North West	2.0	2.3	22,917	24,561	7.2
Yorkshire and the Humber	1.7	2.0	14,615	15,733	7.6
East Midlands	1.8	2.1	12,603	14,327	13.7
West Midlands	1.8	2.2	16,526	18,979	14.8
East of England	1.5	2.0	13,100	17,497	33.6
London	1.9	2.2	22,044	26,231	19.0
South East	1.4	1.9	17,692	24,974	41.2
South West	1.5	2.2	11,883	16,118	35.6

Source: White C., *2011 Census Analysis: Unpaid Care in England and Wales, 2011 and Comparison with 2001*, Office for National Statistics, Wales, UK, 2013.

Time Spent on Caring

The amount of time dedicated to caregiving varies considerably. Table 1.4 outlines the breakdown of unpaid carers by hours of caring from both 2001 and 2011 census data.

It can be seen that the trend here of time dedicated to being a carer is similar across the decade, with a slight increase in 2011 towards carers giving 50 hours or more to unpaid care. What is of note here is that males and females across England and Wales are between two and three times more likely to have poor general health if they provide 50 hours or more unpaid care per week than if they provide no unpaid care (ONS 2013). This finding highlights the huge impact upon health and well-being as a consequence of unpaid caring to this extent. We will cover the impact of caring on carers and family in Chapter 3.

What is important to say here is that as carers often juggle the care they give with their personal and work life and other responsibilities, simply taking a break can be a major challenge. In 2008, the government sought to highlight the plight of carers by publishing a carer's national strategy (DH 2008a) and an influential document 'Carers at the heart of 21st century', making clear that carers need a life of their own (DH 2008b). As seen with young carers (Hounsell 2013), raising the profile, experiences and needs of carers

Table 1.4 Breakdown of unpaid care categories for England and Wales from the 2001 and 2011 census data

Extent of unpaid care	Percentage[a]	
	2011	2001
No unpaid care	89.7	90.0
1–19 hours	6.5	6.8
20–49 hours	1.4	1.1
50 hours or more	2.4	2.1

Source: White C., *2011 Census Analysis: Unpaid Care in England and Wales, 2011 and Comparison with 2001*, Office for National Statistics, Wales, UK, 2013.
[a] Percentages are rounded to one decimal place.

requires more than just illumination and policy rhetoric (Allen 2000); it requires practical application and interventions to address their support needs (Chapter 6 covers nursing interventions).

Gender Differences

In terms of gender, there are some differences across all age groups in both England and Wales – women account for 58% of unpaid carers and men 42%. According to the 2011 census data (ONS 2013), unpaid care provision by age and sex is found to be as follows:

- Unpaid care is highest for both men and women in the 50–64 age range.
- Women provide a higher share across ages 0–64, but men aged 50–64 do provide a higher percentage of unpaid care than women aged 25–49.
- The possibility of becoming an unpaid carer increases up to age 64.
- People in the 50–64 age range are the most likely to have an elderly parent to care for.
- Becoming an unpaid carer in your 50s increases your chances of leaving the labour market for good, is associated with health problems and restricts your social and leisure activities.

These levels of unpaid care undoubtedly contribute to financial savings for health and social care provision within the United Kingdom (2008a). Cost savings to society are underestimated; however, Carers UK in 2011 claimed that carers (relatives or friends) in the United Kingdom save £119 billion a year or almost as much as the entire cost of the National Health Service (NHS). The first estimate of the value of carers was made in 1984, but the first comparable figure, in 1989, put their contribution at £24 billion. Clearly, carers are making a massive contribution to society year on year, and as stated earlier, with the ageing population, greater numbers of severely disabled people living longer and improved management of long-term conditions, caring has become a fact of life for every family.

But many carers are struggling with little or no help or are facing cuts in the services and benefits they rely on. Pickard, in 2008, highlighted that by 2014 the number of people needing care will outstrip the number of people able to provide that care (Pickard 2008). An ageing population, smaller family size and geographic mobility have all contributed to what is a growing crisis for national and local government, the NHS and employers (Buckner and Yeandle 2011).

Awareness of Carers

Historically, nurses and other health professionals have lacked awareness of the major role played by carers. However, efforts to raise awareness and to identify and support carers have been much more consistent since the publication of the UK National Carers Strategy in England (DH 1999, 2010b). This positive attention has been an ongoing process which, according to Hughes et al. (2013, p. 78), has needed 'the force of legislation, though a Private Member's Bill in the UK House of Commons is designed to enhance the identification and support of carers' (which failed to make parliamentary progress [Carers Identification and Support Bill, 2012]). That said, it has been through the UK Carers Act (2014) and the Children and Families Act (2014) that new rights entitle carers and the people they care for to a clear assessment of their needs irrespective of their finances or level of need (Carers Trust 2014). From April 2015, an additional dimension to the carer assessment* was included, that being *whether you are able or willing to carry on caring* (Carers UK 2015).

Complementarily, and interestingly, in 2004, the Quality and Outcomes Framework (QOF) for GP contracts in the United Kingdom made explicit mention for general practitioners (GPs) to have systems in place for identifying and referring carers to local authorities for assessment of their needs (DH 2004). The QOF rewards GPs for their performance in the care of their patients and includes measures for addressing and supporting carers. More recently, the Royal College of Nursing (RCN), in partnership with the UK Department of Health (DH), held four summits in February 2015 aimed at nurses to inspire them to make a difference in the lives of carers. This partnership was part of a carers' project led by the RCN that sought to take forward data from the four summits to key stakeholders, such as ministers, in June 2015. Similarly, The Queen's Nursing Institute (QNI) commenced a dedicated carers' project to raise awareness of carers amongst community nurses (district nurses, school nurses, health visitors, practice nurses and all nurses in community practice settings). The QNI has developed free online resources to support nurses who work with carers and other supportive materials. Clearly, the DH carers' strategy has had an influence here and has sought to underpin the carers' projects at the RCN and QNI (DH 2008a,b). What is important is that within nursing and general practice, recognition of, and support for, carers is very much a high priority throughout the United Kingdom, not simply to signpost carers but to value, respect and care for them too.

NHS provision is in constant need of addressing attitudes and barriers towards carers within its workforce alongside more understanding and awareness of carers' issues. The issues that carers face are too often overlooked, ignored or hidden. Arguably, as health professionals lack awareness, uncertainties can unfold in relation to being able to do anything to support carers and their issues. Inclusion of training within professional education programmes has

---

* A carer's assessment is for adult carers of adults (over 18 years) who are disabled, ill or elderly. It is an opportunity to discuss with your local council what support or services you need. The assessment will look at how caring affects your life, including, for example, physical, mental and emotional needs and *whether you are able or willing to carry on caring* (Carers UK, 2015).

been limited and in some cases non-existent (Greenwood et al. 2010). As authors, we have been mindful of this context and in response we designed in 2009 a specific undergraduate learning module within a preregistration nursing curriculum entitled 'Supporting families and carers'. Our aspirations were to not only raise awareness of caregivers but also equip student nurses with knowledge and understanding of the key issues so as to inform their practice and engagement with families and caregivers in any care setting.

In further support of carers, NHS England (2014) recently published its commitment to carers in a document setting out a series of priorities and commitments to the thousands of carers in England to ensure that their involvement in patients care is valued and respected. Moreover, it sets out its commitments within the UK policy context of the NHS, and it conducted a participation exercise in December 2013 with carers across England. From this work, NHS England said it would deliver and move forward on eight priorities (NHS England 2014, p. 10):

1. Raising the profile of carers
2. Educating, training and providing information
3. Developing services
4. Providing person-centred, well-coordinated care
5. Providing primary care
6. Commissioning support
7. Creating partnerships
8. Making NHS England an employer

Clearly, the visibility, value and active involvement of carers need to be seen and heard in constructive and meaningful ways. To address this, within each of these eight priorities are a set of specific commitments to enable commissioners, managers, service providers, health professionals and the public to guide them towards improving carers' experiences, contributions, inclusion in decisions and presence in caregiving in every aspect of service provision. As we move forward in seeking to attain such priorities and commitments, the UK Carers Act (2014), with its carer assessment rights amended with effect from April 2015, provides huge opportunities to help and support carers and their families. This legal change is considered a welcome landmark by such organisations as Carers UK, as for the first time the option of a carer's assessment moves to an actual requirement, in other words, a 'must do' (Carers Trust 2014).

Caregiving Tasks/Responsibilities

The types of tasks and levels of caregiving are highly variable across the caregiving population. A huge assortment of variables and confound factors come into play dependent upon personal circumstances, which then connect directly to caregiving tasks and responsibilities. Caregiving can be extensive and all-consuming in that 'caring' can take over a carer's life and result in lack of personal freedom. Conversely, at the other end of the spectrum, caregiving may only require the offer of informal social support with minimal direct personal care being required. It is worth mentioning that the relationship between high-level, extensive care tasks and mental health of caregivers is an area of concern notably within the voluntary sector and yet remains under-researched. That said, we will discuss links between intensive or extensive caregiving and the impact upon health and well-being more broadly in Chapters 3 and 4.

We know that caregiving tasks can include activities of daily livings (ADLs), for example, washing and dressing, feeding, toileting and managing incontinence, preparing meals, shopping, providing supervision and managing financial and legal issues. In terms of tasks, ADLs or instrumental ADLs (IADLs) are frequently used as indicators of the functional status of care recipients. However, assisting with ADLs and IADLs does not adequately capture the complexity and stressfulness of caregiving. For example, by their nature, tasks alone do not indicate caregiver workload, i.e., time and energy spent by family member(s) or carers in undertaking their care tasks and responsibilities. The consequences of such tasks and workload can effect caregiver's mood functions, feelings of satisfaction and worth and sense of freedom, thus potentially creating loneliness, depression, isolation and feelings of burden (Reinhard et al. 2008).

Caregiving tasks can be broken down into two distinct areas – direct and indirect tasks, as outlined here:

Direct tasks – physical and practical

- Personal care such as getting in and out of a bed or chair, bathing, dressing, walking, eating, medication administration and toileting
- Household activities such as (1) housework (assistance in making beds, doing laundry, preparing meals, washing up, cleaning and vacuuming) and (2) household maintenance (washing windows, gardening and minor household repairs)
- Shopping and transportation, which includes assistance in shopping and running errands

Indirect tasks – psychosocial

- Financial affairs, such as help with personal banking, paying bills and filling in forms
- Emotional support, which involves assistance in social interaction, providing opportunities for socialisation and managing challenging behaviours and mood swings
- Monitoring care, which includes ensuring that the care recipient's needs are being met and services provided are of an appropriate standard

It is worth pointing out that breaking down caregiving tasks into two distinct areas should not be interpreted as being that straightforward. Caregiving is not that neat and simple; carers and families don't always see these tasks as a workload, but they are often thought of as an integral part of 'caring' for family, friends or neighbours. What can typically happen is that carers move in and out of these direct and indirect tasks with differing skills, knowledge and abilities to manage them. Several family members can be helping out, or not. The impact of carer's workload and unpredictable nature of caring creates 'hassles and pile up' at individual and collective levels (see Chapter 3). Interestingly, the ways in which men and women approach caregiving can be different, with preferences placed upon different tasks. Finch (1990) highlighted how women can be socialised into the 'ethic of care'; consequently, the caring role has tended to be traditionally for women. That said, the trend is changing with more men undertaking caregiving in the United Kingdom (White 2013), although men may engage in tasks different to those of women; typically, the responsibilities in indirect tasks can impact similarly on men and women. Regardless of what can be seen is that such a variable and often unpredictable workload can evolve into a balancing act between caregiving and other activities such as work, family and leisure. Whether this is as a family unit with several family members working together or caring alone, the demands can be physically, socially and psychologically huge.

There is no doubt that different tasks provided by caregivers require different skills and attributes, as the dimension of caregiving tasks are bound up in factors such as

- Nature of tasks
- Frequency with which tasks are performed
- Hours of care provided each day
- Skills, knowledge and abilities of carers to perform the tasks
- Extent to which tasks can be routine, as such incorporated into daily life
- Support available from other family members

Caregivers can feel alone and isolated in their caring roles, depending upon the nature of care recipients' illness severity and needs and may well negatively appraise their caregiving. At the same time, carers can feel supported and manage to cope well. The opportunistic nature of nursing can be important here in that encounters that occur with patients or care recipients provide 'a window of opportunity' into considering the carer. Such encounters can be meaningful and significant in the lives of a carer and family member(s); such opportunities ideally should not be overlooked or undervalued. At this juncture, we suggest that you watch either of these two films (both if you wish), which were made to raise awareness of carers across the life course and to offer insights into ways in which health professionals can play a role:

1. https://www.youtube.com/watch?v=_901EtOAms4 (*Invisible or Ignored* – a documentary made by Young Carers in Salford and The Lowry)
2. https://www.youtube.com/watch?v=zzYkSp9_Tro (a video about the issues relating to caring for someone with mental health problems, produced by GMW Mental Health Foundation Trust)

Thinking Box

These two films are distinctly different but raise pertinent issues for us all in the caring profession.

Make some notes of your thoughts, for example, in terms of

- Specific opportunities for nurses
- Areas you could incorporate into your practice
- Your learnings

We will return to the notion of 'lost opportunities' in Chapter 7, where we discuss working with families and carers in some detail. But for now keep your notes and reflect upon your thoughts.

The tasks, responsibilities and, ultimately, roles of a caregiver undoubtedly change over time and thus so do their experiences. As we know, caregiving can last for a short period of post-acute care, especially after hospitalisation, to more than 40 years of ongoing care for a person with chronic care needs, such as neurological diseases. Perhaps one of the most challenging and frustrating phenomena in the first stages of a carer's 'career' is obtaining an accurate diagnosis. For example, in the case of Alzheimer's disease, this may take several years. The build-up period to securing a diagnosis can be particularly draining in the lives of families as they are likely to have taken on more activities and responsibilities, for example, in the case of progressive degenerative diseases such as multiple sclerosis, Parkinson's disease and dementia. Aneshensel et al. (1995) noted in their work with dementia caregiving the expression 'the unexpected career'. Irrespective of the reasons for caring, typically a caregiving role or career is often unplanned and carer's trajectory can involve a variety of periods of stability, changes and numerous transitions.

In support of understanding the carer journey, Given and Given (1991) refer to the 'natural course' of caregiving and provide four stages that family caregivers go through:

1. Selection into the role
2. Acquisition of care-related skills
3. Provision of care
4. Cessation of care

Undoubtedly, the concept of a *natural course* seems to make sense but does not necessarily follow a sequential process in every case nor capture the personal dimensions of someone's natural course in practice. The most obvious to think about here is perhaps stage 1 – selection into the role – as this could infer choice, consent and perhaps self-selection into the role; of course, this is highly variable in reality. Interestingly, the final stage in Given and Given's natural courses may well result in a positive outcome such as recovery from illness but equally a negative outcome such as death. In support of the natural course concept, other authors such as Aneshensel et al. (1995) and Nolan et al. (2003) remind us of the temporal experience of caregiving to reflect the changing nature of caregiving over time. For nurses, these theoretical ideas are important in considering their role in relation to the iterative nature of assessments and caregiving changes (see the 'Interventions to Support Families and Carers' section in Chapter 6).

As mentioned earlier, a significant factor affecting the provision of informal care in the Western world is the ageing population (UN 2013; WHO 2014). Older people are already involved in large amounts of caregiving responsibilities in modern society, and this trend is set to increase. As individuals age, they increasingly experience limitations in their ability to perform ADLs (e.g. bathing and dressing) as well as IADLs (e.g. driving and paying bills) (Kenneth and Kenneth 2000). Subsequently, many of these elderly individuals depend on assistance from others to perform their everyday activities. Many older carers (such as sandwich carers) often have healthcare problems of their own, increasing their chance of acquiring stress and burden compounded by caring roles.

Deprivation is associated with a higher prevalence of unpaid care (Young et al. 2005), as well as with high levels of illness, poverty, worklessness and social exclusion. Whilst recent advances in health and medicine mean that people with long-term health problems have longer life expectancy and enable a higher proportion of children with chronic poor health or serious disabilities to survive into adulthood, these welcome developments also bring increasing demand for care and carers.

Patterns of carers have changed with advances in modern medicine and medical health research, and now there is an emergence of what has been termed a 'new survivor generation'. With advanced technologies and treatments, the new survivor generation can be anyone but typically consists of children and younger people who survived rare cancers and those (of any age) surviving acquired brain injury (e.g. traumatic brain injury and stroke) who, following treatment, are expected to live a long life. Whereas years ago such people would have died, with advances in modern medicine, life expectancy has improved dramatically for many people in our society. In addition to this medical progress and new survivor generation, we are also seeing what has been termed 'career carers' (see Table 1.1).

Thinking Box

Can you think of someone you have come across who could be regarded as a new survivor generation?

Did you consider the notion of carer in this situation?

What do you think the implications could be for the carer and the survivor?

What could you do in this situation?

Key Points

- The number of 'informal' carers, including young and older carers, will increase significantly in the developed world over the coming years.
- Caregivers are most often spouses or adult children and predominantly women.
- Carers are often elderly themselves.
- A carer may be looking after more than one person.
- The average time span of caring and a carer's role change over time.
- Caregivers perform many tasks which also vary over time, often untrained and lacking in skills to guide their roles.

Chapter Summary

In this chapter, we have provided an overview of the context of carers to raise awareness with regard to their existence, challenges, roles and huge contributions to people's lives. We urge you to watch the three films suggested as they provide insights into many of the issues that carers face. Moreover, they are based on real lives and real people, not fiction but truth and genuineness. We feel they supplement many of the core messages we seek to convey throughout this book and indeed this opening chapter.

There is no escaping the fact that the number of carers is increasing in the United Kingdom and the actual need for carers will also grow. Therefore, as nurses, it is imperative that we understand and have deeper insights into the contextual factors regarding the type of caregiving and temporal nature of caring regardless of whether it is for short terms or for long periods of time. There is of course no 'magic wand' to lighten the load for the vast amount of carers in our society but we must support and respect them. Small things matter, such as acknowledging their existence, involving them in decision-making and working together to implement measures that can help. Building therapeutic relationships and trust is the basis for holistic care for patients, carers and their loved ones. We can all make a difference and we all have a responsibility – 'it is a collective endeavour' supporting carers.

In the following chapters, we explore in some detail the consequences and impact of caregiving on the carer. Before that, Chapter 2 provides an overview of families and some of the theoretical perspectives that are worthy of consideration in supporting families and carers.

References

Agard SA and Maindl HT. (2009) Interacting with relatives in intensive care unit: Nurses perceptions of a challenging task. *British Association of Critical Care Nurses* 14(4): 264–272.

Allen D. (2000) Negotiating the role of expert carers on an adult hospital ward. *Sociology of Health and Illness* 22(2): 149–171.

Alzheimer's Disease International (ADI). (2009) World Alzheimer Report 2010. London, UK: ADI.

Aneshensel CS, Pearlin LI, Mullan JT, Zarit SH and Whitlatch CJ. (1995) *Profiles in Caregiving: The Unexpected Career.* San Diego, CA: Academic Press, Inc.

Benner P, Hooper-Kyriakidis P and Stannard D. (1999) *Clinical Wisdom and Interventions in Critical Care.* Philadelphia, PA: WB Saunders.

Buckner LJ and Yeandle SM. (2011) *Valuing Carers 2011: Calculating the Value of Carers' Support.* London, UK: Carers UK.

Care Act. (2014) The Stationery Office, London, UK. http://www.legislation.gov.uk/ukpga/2014/23/pdfs/ukpga_20140023_en.pdf (accessed 29 June 2015).

Carers Identification and Support Bill, 2010–2012, www.parliament.uk.

Carers Trust. (2014) What is a carer? http://www.carers.org/whats-a-carer (accessed 20 August 2014).

Carers UK. (2011) Caring at a distance: Bridging the gap. http://www.carersuk.org/news-and-campaigns/press-releases/caring-at-a-distance-bridging-the-gap (accessed 29 June 2015).

Carers UK. (2015) Assessments and the Care Act: Getting help in England from April 2015. Factsheet E1029. London, UK: Carers UK. www.carersuk.org.

Children and Families Act. (2014) The Stationery Office, London, UK. http://www.legislation.gov.uk/ukpga/2014/6/pdfs/ukpga_20140006_en.pdf (accessed 29 June 2015).

Chisholm JF. (1989) The sandwich generation. *Journal of Social Distress and the Homeless* 8: 177–180.

Conn L. (2006) *Literature Review to Inform the Inspection of Social Care Support Services for Carers of Older People in Northern Ireland.* Belfast. Northern Ireland: Department of Health, Social Services and Public Safety. http://www.dhsspsni.gov.uk/de/print/oss_literature_review_carers_of_old_people.pdf (accessed 20 August 2014).

Cronin P, Hynes G, Breen M, McCarron M, McMallion P and O'Sullivan L. (2014) Between worlds: The experiences and needs of former family carers. *Health and Social Care in the Community* 23(1): 88–96.

DH. (1999) *Caring about Carers: A National Strategy for Carers.* London, UK: Department of Health.

DH. (2004) *Quality and Outcomes Framework Guidance.* London, UK: Department of Health.

DH. (2008a) *The Carers National Strategy Organisation.* London, UK: Department of Health.

DH. (2008b) *Carers at the Heart of 21st Century Families and Communities: A Caring System on Your Side, A Life of Your Own.* London, UK: Department of Health.

DH. (2010a) *Personalising Services and Support for Carers Organisations*. London, UK: Department of Health.

DH. (2010b) *Recognised, Valued and Supported: Next Steps for the Carers Strategy: Response to the Call for Views*. London, UK: Department of Health.

DH. (2012) *Compassion in Practice: Nursing, Midwifery and Carer Staff: Our Vision and Strategy*. London, UK: Department of Health.

DH. (2013a) *Care in Local Communities: A New Vision and Model for District Nursing*. London, UK: Department of Health.

DH. (2013b) *Helping Carers to Stay Health*. London, UK: Department of Health.

Fengler AP and Goodrich N. (1979) Wives of elderly disabled men: The hidden patients. *The Gerontologist* 19(2): 175–183.

Finch F. (1990) The politics of community care. In: C. Ungerson (Ed.) *Gender and Caring: Work and Welfare in Britain and Scandinavia*. New York: Harvester Wheatsheaf, pp. 34–58.

Given BA and Given CW. (1991) Family caregiving for the elderly. *Annual Review of Nursing Research* 9: 77–101.

Greenwood N, Mackenzie A, Habbi R, Atkins C and Jones R. (2010) General practitioners and carers: A questionnaire survey of attitudes, awareness of issues, barriers and enablers to provision of services. *BMC Family Practice* 11: 100.

Heron C. (1998) *Working with Carers*. London, UK: Jessica Kingsley.

Hounsell D. (2013) *Hidden from View: The Experiences of Young Carers in England*. London, UK: The Children's Society. www.childrenssociety.org.uk.

Hughes N, Locock L and Ziebland S. (2013) Personal identity and the role of 'carer' among relatives and friends of people with multiple sclerosis. *Social Science and Medicine* 96(100): 78–85.

Kenneth GM and Kenneth CL. (2000) Active life expectancy estimates for the U.S. elderly population: A multidimensional continuous-mixture model of functional change applied to completed cohorts, 1982–1996. *Demography* 37: 253.

Laing M and Sprung S. (2013) *Carers Project Literature Review*. London, UK. www.qni.org.uk/docs/Carers_Literature_Review.doc (accessed 12 March 2015).

Lloyd L. (2006) Call us carers: Limitations and risks in campaigning for recognition and exclusivity. *Critical Social Policy* 26(4): 945–960.

Marriott H. (2013) *Selfish Pig: Guide to Caring*, 1st ed. Leominster, UK: Orphans Press.

Molyneaux V, Butchard S, Simpson J and Murray C. (2011) Reconsidering the term 'carer': A critique of the universal adoption of the term. *Ageing & Society* 31: 422–437.

Montogmery R. (1999) The family role in the context of long-term care. *Journal of Aging and Health* 11(3): 383–416.

Montgomery RJV and Kosloski KD. (2000) Family caregiving: Change, continuity and diversity. In: M. P. Lawton and R. L. Rubestein (Eds.) *Interventions in Dementia Care: Towards Improving Quality of Life*. New York: Springer.

NHS England. (2014) *NHS's England Commitment to Carers*. Leeds, UK: NHS England.

Nolan MR, Lundh U, Grant G and Keady J. (Eds.) (2003) *Partnerships in Family Care*. Buckingham, UK: Open University Press.

Norlyk A and Martinsen B. (2013) The extended arm of the health professionals? Relatives experiences of patients recovery in a fast-track programme. *Journal of Advanced Nursing* 69(8): 1737–1746.

NMC. (2001) *Standards for Specialist Education and Practice.* London, UK: NMC.

Parkinson's UK. (2013) http://www.parkinsons.org.uk/content/about-parkinsons.

Perkins EA and Haley WE. (2010) Compound caregiving: When lifelong caregivers undertake additional caregiving role. *Rehabilitation Psychology* 55(4): 409–417.

Perlesz A, Kinsella G and Crowe S. (2000) Psychological distress and family satisfaction following traumatic brain injury: Injured individuals and their primary, secondary and tertiary carers. *Journal of Head Trauma Rehabilitation* 15(3): 909–929.

Personal communication. (2013) Member of a user/carer group in University of Salford, Manchester, England.

Pickard L. (2008) Informal care for older people provided by their adult children: Projections of supply and demand to 2041 in England. Report to the Strategy Unit and Department of Health. Also published as part of 'Tipping Point for Care: Time for a New Social Contract', 2010. London, UK: Carers UK.

Reinhard SC, Given B, Huhtala Petlick N and Bemis A. (2008). Chapter 14: Supporting family caregivers in providing care. In: R. G. Huges (Ed.) *Patient Safety and Quality: An Evidence-Based Handbook for Nurses.* Rockville, MD: Agency for Healthcare Research and Quality (US).

United Nations. (2013) Ageing populations. http://www.un.org/en/development/desa/population/publications/dataset/urban/profilesOfAgeing2013.shtml (accessed 29 June 2015).

White C. (2013) *2011 Census Analysis: Unpaid Care in England and Wales, 2011 and Comparison with 2001.* Wales, UK: Office for National Statistics.

WHO. (2014) Facts about ageing. http://www.who.int/ageing/about/facts/en/ (accessed 29 June 2015).

Young H, Grundy E and Kalogirou S. (2005) Who cares? Geographic variation in unpaid caregiving in England and Wales: Evidence from the 2001 Census. *Population Trends* 120: 23–34.

Useful Links

Carers UK is the United Kingdom's only national membership charity for carers; it is both a support network and a movement for change: http://www.carersuk.org/.

Office for National Statistics (ONS) is the UK's largest independent producer of official statistics and is the recognised national statistical institute for the United Kingdom: http://www.ons.gov.uk/ons/index.html.

QNI is a registered charity dedicated to improve the nursing care of people in their own homes: http://www.qni.org.uk/.

Twitter Accounts
@CarersUK
@CarersTrust

2

The Family

Introduction

This chapter concentrates on the theoretical frameworks pertaining to families and caregivers, including concepts such as functionalism, general systems theory, family systems and different family structures. Definitions of families are offered alongside influencing factors such as motivation, obligation and willingness to undertake the caregiving role. The final section introduces family partnerships and family-centred practice. We feel it is important that nurses understand these concepts and theories as the whole dynamics of society, demographics of families and healthcare is changing. As nurses, we need to understand the implications of how we approach and support families.

In seeking to understand carers and caregivers, we need to understand 'the family'. Throughout history and cultures, families have been the most enduring institutions in the world. As nurses, we engage with families and relatives as part of our everyday practice irrespective of practice context and the nature of illness or health condition. In doing so, we, as nurses, aim to build trust and respect in order to create and sustain good relationships between professionals, patients, families and caregivers. Of course this ambition is not exactly new; for example, nurse theorists such as Jean Watson, Betty Neuman and Joyce Travelbee, to name a few, have articulated the importance of the family within their theoretical frameworks and humanistic nursing models. Likewise in the United Kingdom, the Nursing and Midwifery Council (NMC), which was the United Kingdom Central Council (UKCC) before, has made explicit that inclusion of the family and carer dynamic is embedded within all aspects of nursing relationships in practice. In essence, family and caregivers in the broadest sense of the definition (see the 'Definitions of Carers' section in Chapter 1) are fundamental to holistic nursing care (see salutogenesis in Chapters 3 through 5). Therefore, this chapter offers a more comprehensive understanding of some of the theoretical concepts which we hope you will find useful to inform and support your day-to-day practice.

Context

The family is one of the oldest and most universal of all social institutions. It can exert a powerful influence on individuals in terms of experiences of health and illness, as families play a key role in the nurturing and socialisation of the young and are important as a source of nursing care, caring and information about health and illness.

What is interesting is that the family and its history has been the subject of much research for decades and the literature agrees on one thing: that no single family system exists. In fact,

Murray and Barnes (2012) put forward a broad statement to say that the family is 'a specific blend of social relations that have been constructed and reconstructed in many different forms throughout history' (p. 533).

Whatever the concepts of family are, they tend to mirror economic, political, sociocultural contexts and are reflective of time and place. That said, we do know that the West has always been characterised by diversity of family forms and functions and by diversity of attitudes to family relationships (Davey 1995). In current society, biology or kinship is no longer considered the single determinant of 'family'.

Caregiving and support during times of illness has been at the heart of family life for centuries. Whatever the definition of a family offered in the literature, family members depend on one another especially in times of illness, trauma and injury. The decisions that are made, whether those need medical, nursing or residential care, directly affect the caregiver and the patient. Families affected by an illness trauma or long-term illness ES or disabling conditions can be faced with a raft of relational opportunities and challenges. Challenges include long-standing family roles and patterns of family organisation.

We have seen in nursing discourses and policy the term 'significant others' used to encompass those outside the immediate family who may well be involved in caring for someone and who ought to be included in care planning and decision-making processes. In this sense, families are considered the unit of care; by doing so, Hanson (2005) suggests that nurses have much broader perspectives for approaching healthcare needs of both individual family members and the family unit as a whole. Indeed, research in primary care has shown that good communication skills with shared decision-making and a participatory approach can enhance patient well-being (Ruiz Moral 2010).

As mentioned in Chapter 1, family caregivers may have to relinquish time from work, with economical consequences, in order to carry out their caregiving activities. Informal caregiving often has a considerable impact on women carers' ability to fully participate in paid work (see Chapter 5). Families even vary within given cultures because every family has its own unique culture. People who come from the same family of origin create different families over time. Ethnic/racial background and 'culture' are used synonymously in some sources of the literature to infer that a group of people have shared values, beliefs and ways of being. However, it should not be assumed that because families are from a particular background, their beliefs are similar. People from some groups may or may not express similar needs and priorities. It is important to find out what those needs and priorities are and individualise services to meet their specific needs. That said, we know that notions of familism vary across cultures and may well impact upon individualising care favouring shared decision-making with the family and carers.

Before discussing definitions of family in detail, we would like you to think about your own family and answer these two questions (make some notes):

1. How would you define your family?
2. What are the important elements of your family?

Definitions of a Family

As stated, definitions of a family vary in the literature and change over time depending upon culture, politics, economics and society contexts. However, any definition of a family should include the widely quoted definition offered by Beutler et al. (1989) in which the family is characterised as a unique set of relationships, experiences and characteristics*. That said, what is clear is that almost all societies have a family concept and most people experience a family unit of some description over their lifetime.

In seeking to define a family, we often draw upon literature from other disciplines, e.g., social sciences and psychology. We know that definitions differ by discipline, for example,

- *Legal*: Relationships through blood ties, adoption, guardianship or marriage
- *Biological*: Genetic biological networks amongst people
- *Sociological*: Groups of people living together
- *Psychological*: Groups with strong emotional ties

The word 'family' usually means people related by blood or marriage whether they live together or not and a group of people having a history of life in common. The significance here is that these groups of people have evolved ways of living together, and these ways of living form a structure that governs the way these people behave and feel. That said, definition of 'family' by Chynoweth and Dyer (1991) says, 'a family is a group of people, related by blood or circumstance, which rely upon one another for security, sustenance, support, socialisation and stimulation'.

According to this definition, a family can contain individuals who are related by blood, but also by circumstance. Such circumstances can include, but are not restricted to, children and families who identify themselves as foster families, grandparents who are raising their grandchildren and other situations that involve young children/adults being raised by persons other than their biological parents (e.g. stepchildren). In terms of nursing literature, Hanson (2005, p. 5) refers to family as 'two or more individuals who depend on one another for emotional, physical and economical support. The members of the family are self-defined'.

A *family* has been otherwise defined as follows:

A relatively stable living group, a distinct psychosocial unit, that comprises at least some forms of 'nuclear' family and may include other members not necessarily blood or marriage related.

Klagsburn and Davis (1977, p. 149)

A family is a social system operating through transactional patterns which underpin the family system.

Dulfano (1982, p. 24)

More broadly, in the United Kingdom, the Office for National Statistics (2012) takes the view that 'families are defined by marriage, civil partnership or cohabitation, or the presence of children in the household', implying that a family shares the same living space or home.

Boss (2002, p. 18) argues that a rigid monolithic definition of family prevents the family from problem-solving in times of stress. She prefers a wider, more inclusive definition or what has been referred to as the psychological family based upon the family being a continuing

---

* These are (1) the generational nature and permanence of family relationships, (2) concern with 'total' persons, (3) the simultaneous process of orientation that grows out of familial caregiving, (4) a unique and intense emotionality, (5) an emphasis on qualitative purposes and processes, (6) an altruistic orientation and (7) a nurturing form of governance (Beutler et al. 1989, p. 806).

system of interacting persons bound together by processes of shared ritual and rules even more than by shared biology. Boss (2002, p. 18) goes onto argue that

> As well as unity of interacting personalities, the personalities must have history and future together of shared rituals and rules.

She places as much emphasis upon sharing rituals (e.g. birthdays, weddings, funerals holidays) as on the sharing of genetics.

Another term you may come across is the 'invisible family', which means individuals with no biological, legal or sociologically recognised ties to a person and who can be generally overlooked in the literature. However, what is important is that invisible family members do exist and can be a valuable source of support for the person needing care and reflect the non-biological dimension. Paradoxically, this can be stepfamily members, friends and neighbours. That said, it cannot be assumed that being a family member translates automatically into undertaking caregiving or being a carer. Family dynamics and histrionics (to name but a few factors) exist within all families; as such contextual factors play a major role in dictating carer roles, adaptation and coping (see Chapters 3 and 4). For nurses, it is important to understand that health and illness apply to the individual as well as the unit as both are powerful influences in and on family health.

It is important that nurses are knowledgeable about the theories of families, as well as the structure, function and processes of families, to assist them in achieving or maintaining a state of health and well-being. When families are considered the 'unit of care', nurses have a much broader perspectives for approaching healthcare needs of both individual family members and the family unit as a whole (Hanson 2005). Regardless of whether a family is kin or non-kin, the meaning of family is mostly about 'care and trust' within the context of enduring relationships (Murray and Barnes 2012).

The literature agrees that families vary in structure, function and process and that, above all, families are important to, and for, society. We will now move on to explore family functioning and briefly introduce how families function and cope with caregiving (coping is covered in detail in Chapter 4).

Functionalism and Family Function

In trying to understand family function, it is worth mentioning the concept of 'functionalism' with context to acknowledge early thinking on the origins of family functioning. To start with, functionalism is a sociological perspective created by Emile Durkheim, who believed society was made up of interconnected institutions (e.g. education, family and government) that depended on each other to function. Functionalists see society like the human body in that the body relies on the heart to pump blood to other vital organs like the lungs and brain. In addition, functionalists view society constructed of different interdependent components just like family and education. Therefore, in the same way the human body would cease if the heart stopped, functionalists argue society would stop working properly if the family stopped functioning properly. Functionalists say this would happen because family is an institution in which primary socialisation occurs. Primary socialisation is where younger members of a family are taught society's norms, values and beliefs. Therefore, we can see that family has a function in the social system – or to refer back to the body analogy – and has a positive function in the social body (Parsons 1991).

The family function theory claims that each family performs four main functions, namely sexual, procreative, economic and social. Importantly, it is believed that family problems derive from sudden or unexpected changes in the family's structure or processes; these changes, and problems that may ensue, threaten the family's stability and weaken society. What is important to understand is that functionalists believe that families share common residency, are cooperative and are nuclear in form and that these attributes are universal. In seeking to achieve these main functions, a traditional view and expectation is taken of the family and roles, e.g., the man as 'breadwinner' and the woman (wife) as 'homemaker'. In this context, the family can adapt to its different needs and is equipped to be geographically and socially mobile, together as a unit.

Set within functionalism theory is a dominant and influential theory on family function developed by Talcott Parsons and George Murdock in the 1950s. Parsons argued that socialisation, social equilibrium, social order and functional perquisites were all vital for a society to function properly (Parsons 1951, 1967, 1991). Parson's theory of the family believed that industrial societies were ideally served by the 'nuclear family' (considered conventional or mainstream in today's society) and centred upon two key aspects derived from Freudian theory:

1. Socialisation of children
2. Stabilisation of adult's personalities (role specification)

These two aspects, according to Parsons (and other functionalists), are essential functions for society and if not carried out within the family can create problems for society. Whereas Murdock, based on his research on 250 families in 1949, argued there are four essential family functions: sexual, reproductive, economic and educational. Within these four functions, norms and values are traditional; too much deviation from the norms would negatively impact upon the stability of society at large (Adams and Sydie 2001). In this context, we can see that the nature of family is rigid with clear and distinct traditional roles; aligned to clear boundaries and division of labour between men (power and instrumental) and women (affective role and domestic), both roles are viewed as 'natural'. Thus, family functioning relies upon absolute role clarity of all family members. Parsons put forward the 'warm bath theory,' meaning that the family has the function to bath and sooth the family by 'soaking away worries'. The criticisms on functionalism and family theory are plenty and gathered momentum during the 1970s and 1980s mainly for the narrow view of family (excluding same-sex and single parents) and traditional roles, but also for giving no consideration to diversity or offering any alternatives to family (nuclear is the norm) and for being far too idealistic and optimistic. Alternatives for a family do exist, and we know that the Kibbutz Program Center exists for this very reason, and, of course, we have foster care and children's homes.

Criticism of family theories has been notable from the feminist perspective; of note functionalism, for not taking into account the experience of women in the family, as a function that the family is a locus of inequality and exploitation of women and as social policy that takes account of functionalism that favours men and disfavours women (White et al. 2015). Notably, within functionalism, caring is a role expected of women, undertaken within the privacy of the family and largely ignored. It was widely accepted that the function of women in a family is that they are obliged to care, and as such this primary function is considered to be the 'norm' (Molyneaux et al. 2011). In this context, caring was the sole responsibility of women, and indeed for many, the role was forced upon them as an unpaid obligation (Montogmery 1999). What can be seen is that traditions have evolved under the auspice of functionalism that can be seen in some families even today with regard to roles and divisions of labour within the family context. Paradoxically, there has also been a distancing of the traditional, both nuclear and extended, family structure and yet the family remains the most basic relationship in society and the most powerful collaborator of the nurse.

That said, within some cultures and countries, women remain at the 'hub' of the family, often a feature of strong patriarchal norms, where the role of women is bounded in the assumption and obligation of caring and caregiving. Women often, but not exclusively, play a vital role in supporting family function in this context. It is worth acknowledging how heteronormativity of such families (that 'parents' are naturally heterosexual and this is the only sexual orientation) has been problematised from a range of perspectives (e.g. Wilton 2004; Rondahl et al. 2009). The key author here is Wilton, who has debated extensively how social constructions of sexualities have influenced and shaped gender thinking and cultural 'norming' of sexual orientation within dominant traditional theories of the family.

Key Points

- The family is the most universal and oldest of social institutions.
- Definitions reflect culture, politics, economics and social contexts.
- The family can be kin and non-kin.
- The relationship of family to society is interconnected.
- Concepts of family represent both ideological and practical dimensions.
- Traditional views of family tend to defend heteronormativity and shape gender thinking.

Familism

Interestingly, the concept of 'familism' is arguably a dimension of family function with some possible connections to functionalism whereby the family assumes a position of ascendance over individual interests. Within familism, personal interests and rights of an individual are inferior to the values and demands of the family. In other words, the needs of the family are the most important and come before the needs of 'self' or any single member of the family. A central component of familism is the expectation that children will be the primary caregivers for their parents (Wykle and Gueldner 2010, p. 246). However, different from functionalism, cultural norms within society can dictate whether high or low familism exists. For example, typically, Southern European and Latin American countries have been noted to have high familism (Del-Pino-Casado et al. 2012) as noted in Asian and Middle Eastern countries, but arguably the United Kingdom and United States are thought to be low in familism. In respect of high familism, caring for ageing parents and/or sick family members is a deeply embedded integral value and expectation.

In terms of functionalism, the family is seen as a social institution that exists to undertake essential functions for society. Albeit subtle, 'familism' is seen as a social structure that prioritises the family's needs over individuals'; they both agree that family is crucial to the function of society and is the 'backbone' of any society; if things go wrong with the family, then society is affected alongside the health and well-being of the family members and the family as a structured 'unit'.

Thinking Box

What have you observed about families you have met in terms of family functions?

Have you come across the 'traditional' family roles or features of familism? If not, what kind of families have you met? In terms of theory of family functions, what have you observed?

General Systems Theory

Families exist in complex environments, and their relationships are inextricably connected; its members are part of the whole as well as being individuals, and thus multiple relationships and connections exist. So here, we mention general systems theory briefly, as it is a separate discipline in itself. What needs to be understood is the context by which families are both inter- and intraconnected to one another, as a family unit, community and beyond.

As King (1992) rightly points out, the primary objective of nursing is health: its promotion, maintenance and/or restoration; the care of the sick or injured; and the care of the dying. Therefore, nurses need to understand families and communities as a framework within which nurses make transactions in different environments with health as the primary objective (Norris and Frey 2001). The origins of general systems theory are from the biologist Ludwig Von Bertalanffly, who, in the early part of the twentieth century, sought to set out principles to explain all types of systems in all fields of research (sciences, engineering and social systems). The components of a system theory are (1) goals, (2) structures, (3) functions, (4) resources and (5) decision-making (King 1996, p. 15). All these are thought to govern living systems of which the family is a crucial system in any society.

Briefly, general systems theory believes that the 'whole is different from the sum of its parts', and, therefore, when parts or components are examined separately, the results cannot simply be added in order to determine the whole (Nicholas and Everett 1986, 68).

The most important concept to understand within general systems theory is that the organisational characteristics of the system produce a whole that is greater than the sum of its individual parts (Steinglass 1987, p. 44). Importantly, a family is an example of an open, ongoing, goal-seeking, self-regulating social system in that it shares the features of all systems (Broderick 1993, pp. 36–37).

General systems theory views the family as a multidimensional complexity which has an identity of its own, whilst at the same time it is also dynamic in nature, constantly being submitted to stimuli which provoke changes in its structure (Bowen 1971). According to systems thinking, healthy family functioning requires a degree of flexibility to enable families to face a crisis or stressful event (such as becoming a carer for a sick person) by changing individual roles and transactions between various subsystems in order to re-establish a state of equilibrium or balance (Minuchin and Barcai 1969). If the alliances between family members are too 'rigid', transactions are prevented and conflicts become insoluble. As nurses, we often observe the reactions of families when a family member becomes sick or injured; the family's or carer's capacity to deal with change and adapt can be seen in terms of notions of being 'flexible or rigid'. Of course, it can take some time to adjust and establish balance in the family, or not, with a sick or injured family member (sudden change), and as nurses we often have no idea or prior insights into family dynamics, relationships and inter- and intrapersonal knowledge of an individual family. Indeed families are so complex they are not linear or static, and how they function varies considerably. Thus, we are proposing that families need to be understood within the context of systems, the many layers and functions so as to provide insights to inform and guide nursing practice.

Change and Stability

Systems theory sees living systems as responsive to the interplay of two major forces:

1. A morphogenetic force associated with growth, change, development and a tendency to become organised and more complex over time
2. A morphostatic force (called homeostasis) usually conceptualised as a set of regulatory mechanisms useful in maintaining stability, order and control of system functioning (Steinglass 1987, p. 45)

A system has a characteristic of seeking to keep itself in a state of balance and so is always fluctuating between expressions of change and stability. In order to grow and meet the changing demands, a system has to be able to change and experience balance and equilibrium. In order to change and grow, there has to be a certain amount of security and stability. As a rule, families will often attempt to absorb problems in order to continue functioning as a whole. This predisposition to maintain stability is termed 'homeostasis' (Steinglass 1987). Of course, not all families have the capacity to maintain or achieve these two major forces of being morphogenetic and/or morphostatic and obtain homeostasis. But strong families can achieve and maintain family equilibrium by pulling upon their individual and joint strengths to cope effectively. It is also known that strong families are dynamic and responsive to changing needs, development tasks and challenges; they celebrate success and are keen to learn from their mistakes. Interestingly, strong families tend to have clearly defined roles and boundaries, particularly within their parent–child relationships (Guilfoyle et al. 2011). However, as nurses, we have to look at the bigger picture, whole family system, to understand family functioning.

Family Systems Theory

Family systems theory (or family process) is based upon general systems theory. As Turnbull and Turnbull (2001) highlight, family systems theory is grounded within the greater general systems theory, which states that all living systems are composed of interdependent parts. Family systems theory applies general systems theory to the living unit of the family by emphasising interactions and relationships. In other words, a family is a social system operating through transactional patterns that underpin the family system and their function (Dulfano 1982, p. 24). The family is the way it is because of the people that exist in it, and anything that happens in that family affects everyone. Interactions and personalities matter greatly in family systems theory and concepts such as cohesion, equilibrium, flexibility, structure, rules and boundaries are features within this theory.

Family systems theory states that families can be reluctant to change and strive to achieve balance and homeostasis (Steinglass 1987) if something affects it. The ability to achieve homeostasis has many benefits but not all families can do this naturally or alone. For example, this homeostasis is upset when one member sustains an injury or acute illness. In such cases, a family may need to adjust its rules or dynamics to restore balance and accommodate the changing roles and responsibilities of all family members. This can be problematic as families can become enmeshed in one another with their rules, unwritten boundaries and interactions, as typically they are close and do everything together as a 'unit'. It is thought family systems carry out their tasks through subsystems which are always fluctuating between change and stability (Sieberg 1985). Each individual is a subsystem – so a husband, wife or child and larger subgroupings across generations in a family are subsystems.

Most family systems exist along a continuum between enmeshed and disengaged within family systems thinking. Enmeshed refers to boundaries that are blurred, whereas disengaged refers to boundaries that are rigid where communication is difficult (Sieberg 1985, p. 169). So, it can be seen that deviating from the equilibrium can pose challenges for families if boundaries and functions are not clear and well defined. A highly functional family has clear boundaries and rules so that each member retains their sense of individuality but not at the expense of losing the feeling of belonging to a family. Clear boundaries that offer flexibility enable family cohesion and positive interactions, whereas closed boundaries restrict the processing of feedback and limit interaction with external systems and entities (outside the family unit). A boundary may be evaluated in regard of its tangible flexibility and rigidity. Boundaries that move towards rigidity in response to internal or external crises and relax when the threat has passed may be described as possessing an appropriate blend of rigidity and flexibility (Nicholas and Everett 1986, p. 124). In other words, family stability can be achieved through achieving equilibrium and homeostasis (Steinglass 1987).

Key Points

- Both general systems theory and family systems theory agree that families are inter- and intraconnected to one another, as a unit and within the community and beyond.
- Achieving homeostasis, balance and equilibrium is core to the stability of a 'healthy and strong' family.
- Families exist along a continuum.

Family Structure

As discussed earlier within functionalism, just two types of family structures are considered: nuclear family and extended family. Critics put forward that this view presents a mythical family ideal type – arguably a restricted view and somewhat idealistic perspective that fails to include the diversity of family structures present in today's society (e.g. Wilton 2004). Over the past century, family structure has changed in the United Kingdom and notably over the past 50 years or so, with increasing single parenthood and growth of carers in families (Murray and Barnes 2012). In more tolerant societies, arguably families can be self-defining in their type of structure and have the freedoms to choose how they form as a family structure. That said, there are typically seven types of families seen in contemporary society:

1. Nuclear family
2. Extended family
3. Single-parent family
4. Stepfamily
5. Blended family
6. Childless family
7. Grandparent family

Regardless of type and structure, it is the functions and balance of families that determine their value, capacity to change and homeostasis across their life cycle. Within the realms of being a family caregiver which is the main focus of this book, the type of family structure alone bears no resemblance upon the capacity to adapt and cope with caring (as noted earlier in the section 'Family Systems Theory'). Or indeed, it cannot be assumed that a family caregiver has a choice or is willing to accept the term and role.

Cohesion and Togetherness

Before moving on to look specifically at the 'circumplex model' in relation to family cohesion, the notion of togetherness and cohesion is briefly introduced here (for more discussion, see Chapter 3). We know that living with strains and uncertainties of illness, be it sudden or chronic, and/or a disability can be an enormous challenge. There is no such thing as good timing. We know that the main phases of illness and disease are sudden, chronic or terminal. With each phase, families can have time to come together and, in doing so, can try to work in unity or cohesively, but this journey will not be easy irrespective of whether the family is strong and balanced or not. Feelings of coherence are thought to be best described as a continuous process as opposed to stable or static attributes through which individuals and families cope better with stressors (Orgeta and Lo Sterzo 2013). Possessing a high sense of coherence enables individuals and families to manage the stressors of life, such as caregiving, and to cope successfully together. It is thought that a sense of coherence can be a strong predictor of a carer's quality of life (Ekwall et al. 2007), alongside other attributes such as togetherness, homeostasis, flexibility and adaptability, to mention a few, and such cohesion is a useful concept in understanding the impact of caring and being a caregiver.

Throughout this book, we suggest that such a journey, be it short or long, not be seen as a linear process in that a sequence of event flows from a cause (such as illness and disease) but within the context of entire systems. As it is within systems that families interact as a whole, their routines, stability and pattern of being a family can be faced together.

Circumplex Model

Aligned to understanding cohesion and togetherness is a prominent conceptual model called the 'circumplex model'. Olson et al. (1979) proposed the 'circumplex model' for understanding family systems at a relevant time in the family theory community as they were attempting to bridge theory and practice (Olson 1999) as well as designing a tool for usage in clinical assessment and treatment planning in family therapy. These authors argued that two salient aspects 'cohesion' and 'adaptability' are crucial to understanding family dynamics and functioning. They define 'cohesion' as 'the emotional bonding members have with one another and the degree of individual autonomy a person experiences in the family' (Olson et al. 1979, p. 5). 'Adaptability' is defined as 'the ability of a marital or family system to change its power structure, role relationships, and relationship rules in response to situational and developmental stress' (Olson et al. 1979, p. 12). According to the circumplex model, which is based on family systems theory, balanced levels in both cohesion and adaptability make for the healthiest [strong] family dynamics and functioning. Three dimensions – 'flexibility', 'cohesion' and 'communication' – lay at the heart of the circumplex model. The major issue in this model is that balanced couple and family systems tend to be more functional across the life course compared to unbalanced systems. For example, using the circumplex model, families can be classified as either highly balanced or mid-range or low on cohesion and flexibility. In this assessment, what can be seen is that high scores within all categories of the circumplex model are considered to be in the balanced range and represent healthy family dynamics and functioning. In addition, the circumplex model emphasises the interconnectedness of family members and their behaviours (Olson et al. 1989). In summary, the circumplex model is very useful to assess families and their relationships due to the impact of family stress events, such as becoming a caregiver. The adaptability aspect is covered in more detail in Chapter 3.

Roles and Role Theory

Role theory is a theoretical metaphor concerning our social behaviour and characteristics as human beings. It is suggested that our behaviours can be different and predictable depending on people's respective social identities and situations (Biddle 1986). Role can be described as a set of norms that are organised about a function or a comprehensive pattern of behaviours and attitudes. According to Biddle, role theory concerns itself with 'a triad of concepts: patterned and characteristic social behaviours; parts or identities that are assumed by social participants and scripts or expectations for behaviours that are understood by all and adhered to by performers' (Biddle 1986, p. 68). So at the heart of role theory are expectations, behaviours and identities.

Furthermore, role theory entails the idea that humans act in varying and predictable ways based on the expectations and conditions of the social role they are assuming (Biddle 1986). In a practical sense, this can be seen in the lives and experiences of family caregivers and carers. As previously noted, becoming a family caregiver or carer can be unexpected and one can be reluctant to take on or accept the role. When individuals lack sufficient time and resources to fulfil the obligations associated with each of their roles, 'role overload' can ensue (Goode 1960). Role conflict occurs when the expectations of the various roles an individual holds become incompatible (Biddle 1986). Role overload and role conflict are particularly important when discussing caregiving, for example, in relation to women and adult children caregivers' experience of 'burden' (see Chapter 5).

Role theory has evolved as a framework to help understand the multifaceted nature of caregiving effects on their well-being and health. From this, role enhancement and role strain can emerge as competing views explaining how role involvement affects an individual. Whilst role enhancement states that the individual who adopts more roles is likely to experience greater levels of well-being, role strain argues that multiple roles will lead to negative consequences such as role overload. Role strain was originally conceptualised by Goode (1960, 483), who states that it is 'the difficulty in fulfilling role obligations'. An individual may face different types of role demands and role conflicts that are connected to feelings of role strain in response to carrying out specific obligations. For example, caregiving can present an individual with varying and sometimes conflicting array of role obligations and tasks. Of course, this sense of obligation and taking on the role of 'carer' can change over time.

According to role strain theory, the individual will try to make these demands manageable and try to reduce role strain when the caregiver's resources are outstripped and role strain ensues. Competing roles can impact upon a person's willingness to undertake caregiving and actually be a caregiver. As discussed, *being* a carer is compounded by multiple factors such as uncertainties of an illness or disability, which in terms of roles are then 'placed on top of' preexisting roles and relationships, i.e., they are additional roles. Interestingly,

Perkins and Haley (2010) found that in the case of compound carers (see Table 1.1) once past a 'threshold' of caregiving duties, any additional hours or roles are not associated with role strain or distress. That said, huge variation exists and there is no getting away from underestimating role transition, e.g., from son to carer or daughter to carer, the care that is expected to be provided as a carer is incongruent with the role of a son or daughter. This incongruence has the potential to cause distress and strain on the individual who is experiencing changes in his or her role identity. There can be a misconception that family caregivers have adapted a 'healthy' caring role, but as we mentioned earlier, family caregiving is profoundly complex.

For those caregivers who adopt many roles, for example, female caregivers who maintain care within their own family whilst at the same time continue employed work and care also for their elderly parent, role identity and transition, are challenging and particularly relevant. Within families, existing roles are often aligned to skill sets and occupations. For example, health professionals, such as nurses, make connections between their personal and professional lives whereby their skill set is used in a caring context (Manthorpe et al. 2012). Interestingly, Andren and Elmstahl (2005) found, in their study, that family caregivers of persons with dementia reported both moderate burden and great caregiving satisfaction at the same time. These multiple roles may result in role tensions or strains, reduced energy and increased stress. However, multiple roles may provide benefits such as heightened self-esteem, sense of reward and self-efficacy (Del-Pino-Casado et al. 2011a,b).

Thinking Box

Can you identify the multiple roles a family member or carer that you have recently looked after has? Make notes.

Reluctance

Caregivers who are reluctant to care or feel that they have little choice in caregiving face a greater risk of caregiving burden and poor caregiving outcomes (Nolan et al. 1996). The willingness to care cannot be assumed and for some there is reluctance to take on the role and its associated responsibilities. The concept of 'caregiving reluctance' according to Burridge et al. (2007) is an unrecognised and uncommon area of research. Caregiving reluctance has been defined as resistance, aversion or oppositional thoughts or feelings related to the decision to provide care (Burridge et al. 2007). This reluctance may be hidden from others as carers may not readily disclose their feelings as this questions society's norms and expectations. On the one hand, it could be argued that reluctance could be a natural response to becoming a carer, in particular when it is sudden and unexpected. However, caregiver reluctance may not be easily recognised or it may be concealed by other dominating factors such as conflict, financial strain, obligation or social expectation. In their review of the issue, Burridge et al. (2007) clearly demonstrated that whether covert or overt, the impact of caregiving reluctance can be underestimated.

As mentioned, the quality of the relationship before the role of caring can influence the willingness to care. For example, in poor carer–recipient relationships, there may be an unwillingness to care. Thus, willingness to care may be a reflection of the reciprocity and highlights the need to not assume that all families are functional. Reluctance to care can have serious consequences for the health of the caregiver and the care recipient. Thus, what is important is that the consequences of caregiving reluctance require thoughtful consideration by health professionals.

Obligation and Willingness

Feelings of duty or obligation to care can be strong and powerful within families. Often factors such as family history, geographical location, family size and other role responsibilities influence the expectations of providing care. This sense of duty or obligation to care often arises due to a desire to 'give back' or reciprocate past support or is in response to pressure from societal norms (Camden et al. 2011). Pressures versus willingness to care can pose real challenges within families and, from our knowledge, are not fully understood in terms of research studies. What we do know is that cultural norms, such as familism or filial devotion, and societal norms and expectations play a strong role in who cares within a family and subsequently the types of tasks to be performed. The nature of those receiving care in relation to their involvement or decision-making processes in choosing who cares for them is less understood and is worth considering in terms of impact (see Chapter 5). In an ideal world, the carer's relationship would be one way of providing care associated with *willingness* based upon a positive 'healthy and strong' pre-existing relationship mitigated by attributes such as love, generosity and competence to care. However, as we have pointed out, carers often undertake caregiving in the context of adversity, and the consequences of this can be many, all of which are discussed in Chapters 3 through 5.

Motivation to Care

Connected to willingness or obligation are motivations and reasons to providing care, which, for the most part, are inclined to be assumed rather than understood in terms of the literature (Camden et al. 2011). People's motivators to becoming a carer are variable; of course, they could be motivated by emotions such as love, guilt, feelings of obligation, responsibility and closeness and also characteristics such as friendliness, compassion, kindness, appreciation, generosity and a desire to be altruistic. Equally, motivators exist that deter from caring, i.e., to not help, for example, in response to past negative experiences of caring or lack of skills and resources needed to provide care.

Interestingly, 30 years ago, in the context of UK public policy for older people and long-term conditions, Doty (1986) suggested that three primary factors served as motivators to care:

1. Love and affection towards the individual
2. A sense of gratitude and desire to reciprocate past help and caregiving
3. Societal norms of spousal and filial responsibilities

We are not suggesting that these attributes have to be present or are necessary. Indeed, affection, for example, could be missing as a motivator but may not dissuade from caring nor interfere with the quality of caring. Altruistic motivators are thought to be related to early stages of caregiving where feelings of empathy are shown to the care recipient, whereas in the later stages of caregiving, in response to health deterioration or decline of cognitive functions, caregivers can become more egotistically motivated, in other words more self-serving (Quinn et al. 2010). It could be that egotistic motivators are driven by fears of guilt or punishment for not caring or are bound up in the desire for rewards. Feeney and Collins (2003) suggest that people who have egotistic motivations are more likely to provide poor levels of care.

As mentioned, social norms can influence those who take on the role of carer, as kin relationships can determine motivation with spouses most likely to provide care in Western cultures, followed by adult children. Where there is more than one adult child, there is often an expectation that a daughter will provide the care (Quinn et al. 2010). We also know that motivations and expectations can vary in different ethnicities due, in part, to religion and familism or filial commitment (Del-Pino-Casado et al. 2011a). A research study of dementia family caregivers by Romero-Morena et al. (2010) found that fewer personal reasons and more external pressures motivated them to give care.

There is no doubt that motivations to care, from the very outset and over time, can be affected by the nature of the illness or disease alongside perceptions of the challenges that caring could or will bring. That said, it is thought that besides motivation, commitment theory offers insights into one's commitment to both provide and continue to care. In brief, three commitments, namely personal, moral and structural (social pressures or lack of alternatives), are thought to influence one person's commitment to another (Johnson et al. 1999).

Abandonment of the Caregiving Role

For some caregivers, the relationship with the person may become so uncomfortable and strained that they eventually decide to 'abandon' the caregiver role or place their loved one in an institution such as a care home. It is also important to note that some family members are unwilling or unable to become a primary family caregiver. Even for those carers who assume the caregiving role, the question of whether to remain in that role may resurface periodically especially when they are faced with a crisis. For some, the relationship may not be strong enough or the stress may be too great for their coping resources, i.e., the costs of the relationship outweigh the motivation to stay. Capacity to explore other care options is highly dependent upon support and resources, of which economics is the main issue.

Key Points

- Caregiving is affected by a sense of motivation, obligation and willingness.
- Nature of illness and disease, culture, ethnicity and notions of familism all are key factors in providing care.
- At the heart of role theory are expectations, behaviours and identities.

Family Partnerships

Patients and their families do not wish to be passive recipients of healthcare provision but to work in partnership with nurses (DH 1999). It has been suggested that the term 'partnership' denotes a formalised approach, something that emanates from policy and legislation, whilst collaboration is a more active, practice-led process of 'partnership in action' (Whittington 2003, p. 6). Carnwell and Buchanan (2005) add that 'partnership' is an entity, an arrangement or how something is, whereas 'collaboration' is an activity, or what people do. Furthermore, partnership working is also seen as being able to embrace all levels across the range of activities in practice, including engagement and inclusion of the family.

From our experience and knowledge base, true partnerships in care require professionals to view carers (family or not; see the section 'Definitions of the Family') as equal (key) decision-makers. A family partnership approach in healthcare can provide greater capacity for understanding an illness and disease rather than the classic biomedical model (McDaniel et al. 1990). However, the reality of partnerships, decision-making and planning around mutually agreed goals shared between family caregivers and professionals may not always be reflected in practice (Walker and Dewar 2001). Rapport and communication that seek to yield and sustain 'true partnerships' need to be informed and understood with the knowledge base of family systems theory, family structure cohesion and role theory. Given that families are dynamic and unique, professionals need to build partnerships with families, in particular multiple relationships involving individual family members and the family 'collective'. We are not suggesting that this goal is easy, but quite the opposite – it can be demanding and overwhelming. An area of complexity that is particularly challenging concerns the drawing of boundaries between accessing information about the family that enables facilitation of family goals and the family's rights and needs to privacy (Keen and Knox 2004). In Chapter 7, we discuss some of the opportunities that can be useful to support this concern. Of course, harnessing mutual respect and trust from the outset of meeting families and carers provides a solid platform by which to build partnerships. We will return to partnerships in Chapter 7, where we discuss working with families.

Family-Centred Practice

Increasingly, it is recognised that using a family-centred practice is an important consideration when providing services to families living with chronic health problems and disabilities. The term 'family-centred practice' represents a set of beliefs, attitudes and principles that guide the delivery of services to young children with special needs and their families (Bruder 2000, 2001). There is also the belief that the family's priorities should be the guiding force in service delivery (Bruder 2000; Turnbull and Turnbull 2001).

In a diverse culture, such as in the United Kingdom, it is important to recognise that healthcare providers bring values and beliefs to early intervention situations and that culture cannot be left out of the family-centred practice. In some cases, the nurse will be looking at broader goals, whilst the family caregiver may be looking at smaller issues. In cases where families are from a background different from the nurses who are providing the services, this may become problematic. Even when diversity is recognised, it may still be difficult to provide inclusive healthcare due in part to competing tensions for professionals that constrain the extent to which they are willing or able to involve carers (Walker and Dewar 2001). Getting to know the patient by using carers can undermine a nurse's professional identity (Allen 2000). Reaching out to include families and carers in an active role requires time and negotiation skills to be able to break down barriers and create an open sense of space for mutual dialogue.

There is an increasing focus on the research that addresses the needs of families from specific cultural backgrounds. As family's sources of support may be cultural, economic, social or spiritual, early intervention needs to recognise that these types of support may already exist. In addition, it is important that nurses are aware of how these sources may influence the support required to meet their individual needs. For example, the perceived needs of families living in rural areas may be different from those living in urban areas. Researchers have documented that urban and rural factors significantly affect the way services are delivered to families.

The origins of family-centred care are rooted in the historical movement that took place in the early part of the twentieth century to address children's separation from their parents during hospitalisation (Davies 2010). It is incredible to think that children of all ages were subjected to this deeply paternalistic practice and that , as a consequence, the children and parents suffered the impact of separation. It is likely that their memory of this experience remains significant and has shaped their life and relationships. Nowadays, family and relatives play a major role in the hospitalisation of children and adults. In brief, family-centred care (FCC) theory is

> ...an innovative approach to planning, delivery and evaluation of healthcare, governed by mutually beneficial partnerships between the health professional, patient and family
>
> – Institute for Patient- and Family-Centred Care (2010)

Five principles underpin FCC: Dignity, respect, information sharing, participation and collaboration (Tobiano et al. 2012). As nurses, we understand that applying such principles in the context of an FCC approach can result in improved family, caregivers and patient satisfaction. Sadly, however, there is growing evidence to show that although FCC offers an ideal approach to nursing practice, it is not being implemented well into clinical practice settings (Tobiano et al. 2012). Of course, the five principles are recognisable within contemporary healthcare policy and underpin nursing codes of practice (NMC 2015); thus, maybe the idiosyncratic nature of FCC theory is integrated or embedded within different guises. Family-centred care and nursing have developed a body of work within the literature, including research, international and national policies, a critical mass of global experts and many book authors on the subject.

Thinking Box

How in today's healthcare setting do we enable family-centred care?

Key Points

- Theoretical concepts such as functionalism, general systems theory and family systems theory offer insights into understanding families.
- The family is the oldest and most universal social institution, although definitions have changed over time.
- Factors impacting family equilibrium and stability such as illness, disease or disability require the ability to deal with change and test a family's cohesion and togetherness.
- Insights into behaviours towards caregiving have been briefly explored by looking at role theory.
- Motivations towards becoming a carer or caregiver are varied with obligation and willingness alongside notions of familism being strong drivers.
- An overview of family partnerships and family-centred practices was presented.

Chapter Summary

Throughout this chapter, we have been mindful of the vast amount of literature on families, notably in the fields of sociology and psychology; therefore, in respect of this body of work, an overview of the theoretical concepts is offered. What we hope is that you will advance your understandings of the dynamics of families in terms of their presence and involvement (or not) in your role as a nurse. Having a backdrop to the theoretical concepts can go some way to understanding how families react and behave in times of change and strain when faced with health breakdown. As we know, in some families, adjustment, emotions and behaviours can be cohesive and balanced, while in others it can be far more complex. Throughout this chapter, we have avoided the terms 'dysfunctional' or 'functional' due to the tendency to oversimplify their meanings, as disturbance in family equilibrium is multilayered with consequences (more detail in subsequent chapters). How a family functions, on the one hand, is deeply personal and private; however, as we know, with ill health requiring professional involvement, families 'go public'. It is in this context and public arena that we engage with differences in families and their functions and how they manage together, or not, in adapting and coping with their changed health status. In Chapter 3 and 4, we present more details through which we understand adaption and coping.

References

Adams BN and Sydie RA. (2001) *Sociological Theory*. Thousand Oaks, CA: Pine Forge.

Allen D. (2000) Negotiating the role of expert carers on an adult hospital ward. *Sociology of Health and Illness* 22(2): 149–171.

Andrén S and Elmståhl S. (2005) Family caregivers' subjective experiences of satisfaction in dementia care: Aspects of burden, subjective health and sense of coherence. *Journal of Caring Sciences* 19(2):157–168.

Beutler I et al. (1989) The family realm: Theoretical contributions for understanding its uniqueness. *Journal of Marriage and the Family* August: 805–816.

Biddle B. (1986) Recent developments in role theory. *Annual Review of Sociology* 12: 67–92.

Boss P. (2002) *Family Stress Management: A Contextual Approach*, 2nd ed. Thousand Oaks, CA: Sage Publications Inc.

Bowen M. (1971) The use of family theory in clinical practice. In J. Haley (Ed.), *Changing Families*. New York: Grune and Stratton.

Broderick CB. (1993) *Understanding Family Process*. Newbury Park, CA: Sage Publications Inc.

Bruder MB. (2000) Family centred early interventions: Clarifying our values for the new millennium. *Topics in Early Childhood Special Education* 20(2): 105–115.

Bruder MB. (2001) Infants and toddlers: Outcomes and ecology. In: M. J. Guralnick (Ed.) *Early Childhood Inclusion: Focus on Change*. Baltimore, MD: Paul H. Brookes.

Burridge L, Winch S and Clavarino A. (2007) Reluctance to care: A systematic review and development of a conceptual framework. *Cancer Nursing* 30(2): E9–E19.

Camden A, Livingston G and Cooper C. (2011) Reasons why family members become carers and the outcome for the person with dementia: Results from the CARD study. *International Psychogeriatrics* 23(9): 1442–1450.

Carnwell R and Buchanan J. (Eds.) (2005) *Effective Practice in Health and Social Care: A Partnership Approach*. London, UK: Open University Press.

Chynoweth JK and Dyer BR. (1991) *Strengthening Families: A Guide for State Policymaking.* Washington, DC: Council of Governors' Policy Advisors.

Davey B. (1995) Chapter 1: The life course perspective. In: B. Davey (Ed.) *Birth to Old Age: Health in Transition.* Oxford, UK: Open University Press.

Davies R. (2010) Marking the 50th anniversary of the Platt Report: From exclusion, to toleration and parental participation in the care of the hospitalized child. *Journal of Child Health Care* 14(1): 23.

Del-Pino-Casado R, Cold-Osuna A and Moral Palomino PA. (2011a) Subjective burden and cultural motives for caregiving in casual caregiver of older people. *Journal of Nursing Scholarship* 43(3): 282–291.

Del-Pino-Casado R, Cold-Osuna A, Moral Palomino PA and Martinez-Riera JR. (2012) Gender differences regarding informal caregivers of older people. *Journal of Nursing Scholarship* 14(4): 349–357.

Del-Pino-Casado R, Cold-Osuna A, Moral Palomino PA and Pancorbo-Hidalgo PL. (2011b) Coping and subjective burden in caregivers of older relatives: A quantitative systematic review. *Journal of Advanced Nursing* 67(11): 2311–2322.

Department of Health. (1999) *Making a Difference: Strengthening the Nursing, Midwifery and Health Visiting Contribution to Health and Health Care.* London, UK: Stationery Office.

Doty PD. (1986) Family care of the elderly: The role of public policy. *The Milbank Quarterly* 64: 34–75.

Dulfano C. (1982) *Families, Alcoholism and Recovery.* Center City, MN: Hazeldon.

Ekwall AK, Sivberg B and Hallberg IR. (2007) Older caregivers' coping strategies and sense of coherence in relation to quality of life. *Journal of Advanced Nursing* 57: 584–596.

Epstein NB, Baldwin LM and Bishop DS. (1983) The McMaster family assessment device. *Journal of Marital and Family Therapy* 9: 171–180.

Feeney BC and Collins NL. (2003) Motivations for caregiving in adult intimate relationships: Influences on caregiving behavior and relationship functioning. *Personality and Social Psychology Bulletin* 29: 950–968.

Goldenberg I and Goldenberg H. (2008) *Family Therapy: An Overview,* 7th ed. Belmont, CA: Brooks/Cole.

Goode WJ. (1960) A theory of role strain. *American Sociological Review* 25: 483–496.

Guilfoyle S, Goebel J and Pai ALH. (2011) Efficacy and flexibility impact perceived adherence barriers in pediatric kidney post-transplantation. *Families, Systems, & Health* 29(1): 44–54.

Hanson SM. (2005) Family heath nursing: An introduction. In: S. M. Hanson (Ed.) *Family Health Care Nursing: Theory, Practice and Research,* 2nd ed. Philadelphia, PA: F.A. Davies, pp. 3–33.

Institute for Patient- and Family-Centred Care. (2010) http://www.ipfcc.org/faq.html (accessed 8 June 2015).

Johnson MP, Caughlin JP and Huston TL. (1999) The tripartite nature of marital commitment: Personal, moral, and structural reasons to stay married. *Journal of Marriage and Family* 61: 160–177.

Keen D and Knox M. (2004) Approach to challenging behaviour: A family affair. *Journal of Intellectual & Developmental Disability* 29(1): 52–64.

King IM. (1992) King's theory of goal attainment. *Nursing Science Quarterly* 5(1): 19–26.

King IM. (1996) The theory of goal attainment in research and practice. *Nursing Science Quarterly* 9(2): 61–66.

Klagsbum M and Davis DI. (1977) Substance abuse and family interaction. *Family Process* 16: 149–173.

Manthorpe J, Samsi K and Rapaport J. (2012) When the profession becomes personal: Dementia care practitioners as family caregivers. *International Psychogeriatrics* 24(6): 902–910.

McDaniel SH, Campbell TL and Seaburn D. (1990) *Family Oriented Primary Care: A Manual for Medical Providers*. New York: Springer-Verlag.

Minuchin S and Barcai A. (1969) Therapeutically induced family crisis. In J. H. Masserman (Ed.), *Science and Psychoanalysis* (Vol. 14). New York: Grune and Stratton.

Molyneaux V, Butchard S, Simpson J and Murray C. (2011) Reconsidering the term 'carer': A critique of the universal adoption of the term. *Ageing & Society* 31: 422–437.

Montogmery R. (1999) The family role in the context of long-term care. *Journal of Aging and Health* 11(3): 383–416.

Morgan DHJ. (1975) *Social Theory and the Family*. London, UK: Routledge & Kegan Paul.

Murray L and Barnes M. (2012) Have families been rethought? Ethics of care, family and 'whole family' approaches. *Social Policy and Society* 9(4): 533–544.

Nicholas WC and Everett CA. (1986) *Systemic Family Therapy: An Integrated Approach*. New York: Guilford Press.

NMC. (2015) *The Code: Professional Standards of Practice and Behaviour for Nurses and Midwives*. London: Nursing and Midwifery Council. http://www.nmc.org.uk/.

Nolan M, Grant G, and Keady J. (1996) *Understanding Family Care*. Buckingham: Open University Press.

Norris DM and Frey MA. (2001) King's interacting systems framework and theory in nursing practice. In M.R. Alligood and A. Marriner-Tomey (Eds.), *Nursing Theory: Utilization and Application*. London: Mosby, pp. 173–183.

Olson DH. (1999) Circumplex model of marital and family systems. In: F. Walsh (Ed.) *Normal Family Processes*, 2nd ed. New York: Guildford Press.

Olson DH, Sprenkle DH and Russell CS. (1979) Circumplex model of marital and family systems: 1. Cohesion and adaptability dimensions, family types, and clinical application. *Family Process* 18(1): 3–27.

ONS. (2012) *Families and Households, 2001 to 2011; Statistical Bulletin*. London: Office for National Statistics. http://www.ons.gov.uk/ons/dcp171778_251357.pdf (accessed 22 June 2015).

Orgeta V and Lo Sterzo E. (2013) Sense of coherence, burden, and affective symptoms in family carers of people with dementia. *International Psychogeriatrics* 25(6): 973–980.

Parsons T. (1951) *The Social System*. New York: Free Press.

Parsons T. (1991) *Social Systems*. London, UK: Routledge.

Perkins EA and Haley WE. (2010) Compound caregiving: When lifelong caregivers undertake additional caregiving role. *Rehabilitation Psychology* 55(4): 409–417.

Quinn C, Clare L and Woods RT. (2010) The impact of motivations and meanings on the wellbeing of caregivers of people with dementia: A systematic review. *International Psychogeriatrics* 22(1): 43–55.

Romero-Morena R, Marques-Gonzalez M, Losada A and Lopez J. (2010) Motives for caring: Relationship to stress and coping dimensions. *International Psychogeriatrics* 23: 573–582.

Rondahl LG, Bruhner E and Lindhe J. (2009) Heteronormative communication with lesbian families in antenatal care, childbirth and postnatal care. *Journal of Advanced Nursing* 65(11): 2337–2344.

Ruiz Moral R. (2010) The role of physician-patient communication in promoting patient-participatory decision making. *Health Expectations* 13: 33–44.

Sieberg E. (1985) *Family Communication. An Integrated Systems Approach*. New York: Gardner Press Inc.

Steinglass P. (1987) *The Alcoholic Family*. New York: Basic Books Publisher.

Tobiano G, Chaboyer W and McMurray A. (2012) Family members' perceptions of the nursing bedside handover. *Journal of Clinical Nursing* 22: 192–200.

Turnbull AP and Turnbull HR. (2001) *Families, Professionals, and Exceptionality: Collaborating for Empowerment*, 4th ed. Upper Saddle River, NJ: Merrill/Prentice-Hall.

Walker E and Dewar BJ. (2001) How do we facilitate carers' involvement in decision making? *Journal of Advanced Nursing* 34(3): 329–337.

White JM, Klein DM and Martin TF. (2015) *Family Theories: An Introduction*. Los Angeles, CA: Sage.

Whittington C. (2003) *Learning for Collaborative Practice with Other Professions and Agencies*. London, UK: Department of Health.

Wilton T. (2004) *Sexual (Dis)orientation: Gender, Sex, Desire, and Self-Fashioning*. New York: Palgrave Macmillan.

Wykle ML and Gueldner SH. (2010) *Aging Well: Gerontological Education for Nurses*. Sadbury, MA: Jones & Bartlett Learning.

3

Adjusting and Adapting to Caregiving

Introduction

This chapter explores the process of adjusting and adapting to the role of caregiving. We begin by exploring the notion of stress from both individual and family perspectives with an overview of traditional stress and family stress theories. There are a number of theoretical frameworks that can provide a useful means of understanding the stress that results from caregiving. These frameworks help us to understand how carers adjust and adapt to stressors and crisis situations. Traditional stress process theories emphasise the importance of the caregivers' personal and environmental resources in their adjustment, and overall health and mental well-being. Our purpose is not to provide a complete description of the underpinning theories but to outline key theories and their origins in relation to caregiving to help our understanding of adaptation and adjustment processes. Notions of adapting and adjusting will be explored alongside connected theories, notably major family stress and adaptation models, such as the ABCX model and family adjustment and adaptation response (FAAR) model. The concept of resilience is discussed, explaining why some family caregivers are more able to adapt and adjust to their caring role than others is discussed.

Adaptation and Adjustment

One of the complexities in grasping, coping, adjusting and adapting is being clear about what these terms actually mean. So before we begin the discussion on stress, it is necessary to clarify the meaning of terms 'adjustment' and 'adaptation', as often there is a lack of clarity and consistency in the literature. Indeed some authors use the terms interchangeably; however, we suggest there are distinct but subtle differences between them.

Adjustment

The adjustment phase reflects perceived ability to maintain and perform family functions and effective communication when faced with stressors. Where a family caregiver perceives a stressor to be manageable, there is a greater opportunity for healthier adjustment. Adjustment is defined as successful coping which results in effective functioning. For some theorists, adjustment is a short-lived response and adaptation represents longer-term changes that occur in the family (McCubbin and Patterson 1982). Thus, as families adjust to their new circumstances, movement into a more long-term phase adaptation occurs.

Adaptation

Family adaptation is perhaps a more difficult concept to understand and has been explored by several researchers (McCubbin and Patterson 1983a; Boss 2002). Adaptation seems to define the entire process that occurs in response to the stress of caring and relates to the outcome of the adjustment process. It is not a finite end product; rather, it is a continuous process and refers to long-term changes in the family over time, for example, the altering of one's behaviour to meet the demands of the stressor. More specifically, McCubbin and McCubbin (1993, p. 37) define adaptation as

a process in which families engage in direct responses to the extensive demands of a stressor and realize that systemic changes are needed within the family unit to restore functional stability and improve family satisfaction and wellbeing.

Adaptation here refers to the relationships between external demands and the individual's resources and involves changes to family relationships to re-establish both individual and family balance and harmony. Boss (2002) prefers to use the term 'manage' rather than 'adapt' to describe the family's response to stress or crisis, as she states, '...managing high stress and being resilient are indeed the alternative to falling into crisis (p. 89)'. According to Boss (2002), when a family faces a challenging situation that threatens the normal family function, it can lead to temporary family crisis, which means that the family needs to make changes and adapt in order to restore family function. Family adaptation represents the balance between the demands and capabilities of the carer with the demands of the family and community contexts. Central to Olson et al.'s circumplex model, discussed in Chapter 2, is adaptability, defined as

the ability of a marital or family system to change its power structure, role relationships, and relationship rules in response to situational and developmental stress.

Olson et al. (1989, p. 12)

According to Olson et al. (1989), a family's adaptability can be seen as a continuum of the family capacity to change in response to stressors from flexible to rigid or chaotic. This continuum ranges from optimal bonadaptation (positive mental and physical health adaptation) when a stressor causes changes in the family, i.e., adjustment and adaptation, to the negative end of the continuum maladaptation that occurs when families lack resources or strength to adjust and adapt to a state of crisis. For example, a family whose son has survived a traumatic brain injury with severe physical and mental disabilities creates intense caregiving demands, which may be beyond their capabilities, creating stress and maladaptation. According to family systems theory, adaptability is key. All families need to relate to each other in order to grow; adaptation reduces disruption to the family system, restores equilibrium and produces new patterns of functioning. Also emphasised within Olson et al.'s (1989) circumplex model and family systems theory is flexibility of families, as we saw in Chapter 2. Flexibility refers to the ability of families to adjust to new realities by organising themselves and is described as having four levels: chaotic, flexible, structured and rigid. It is the extremes, i.e., rigid and chaotic, that are regarded as being problematic for families. Families who can identify and examine different actions when life throws them challenges, for example, family illness and/or trauma, negotiate a change and are flexible and adaptable. Conversely, families who are unable to see or are unwilling to examine alternative solutions lack flexibility and adaptability. Arguably, these families would benefit from learning problem-solving skills, which we will discuss in more detail in Chapters 4 and 5.

McCubbin and Patterson (1983a) highlight several factors that influence the ability to adjust and adapt, and these include the nature, duration and number of stressors; the family's capabilities and resources to adjust to the demands; and the family's ability to seize the opportunity to produce a change. The stress on family carers may be reduced by a number of available resources, including cohesion, supportive communication, flexibility and other social resources outside the family (McCubbin and McCubbin 1996). In addition, other influences have been identified, for example, family caregiver's spiritual well-being, coping strategies and the relationship between caregiver and care recipient. According to Boss (2002), family appraisal of the situation is a critical variable in the family's adaptation process. Boss (2002) goes on to suggest that the most important component of positive adaptation is how one perceives life stressors and demands.

Key Points

- Adjustment requires short-term changes.
- Adaptation to stressors is a long-term process.
- Adaptation requires significant resources.

Stress and Caregiving

Stress is a highly subjective experience and also a difficult concept to define despite being widely acknowledged. In the literature, many definitions of stress exist and it has been associated with meanings such as hardship, adversity and affliction. Stress can be defined as a stimulus and an observable response to the stimulus. It can be viewed as the negative feelings of being unable to control or manage the problems and external events that occur in everyday life. Three major sources of stress are identified in the literature – life events (relatively rare, which require some significant adjustment), chronic stress or strain (stressors that build slowly and are continuous) and daily stressors or *hassles*, which refer to the micro-interactions in daily life that are irritating and frustrating, such as misplacing things. Carers may experience all three major sources of stress alongside frustrations and conflicts that may arise due to competing demands, needs or goals in caregiving.

Of course, stress is associated with everyday life, and all families, irrespective of gender, culture or ethnicity, experience stress as a result of change. However, within the concept of caregiving, whether this is short term or long term, caregivers may experience many stressful circumstances and events in their caregiving career. Often, carers can be expected to function in this role for many years during which time stressors may challenge their physical and psychological resources. Caregiving stress, like any stressor, can be considered a psychological situation in which the extent of stress is based on the caregiver's perception of the stressful situation, the nature of interactions in the caregiving situation and the individual's personal and environmental resources. Aneshensel et al. (1995) defined stressors in the context of caregiving as 'the problematic conditions and difficult circumstances experienced by caregivers'. These stressors demand adaptation by the caregiver and result in a stress reaction that is highly variable.

Family stress can be viewed as a disturbance in the steady state or equilibrium of the family system, arises from actual or potential stressors and is highly individual and variable depending upon the event or situation. More specifically, family stress, as defined by Boss (2002, 2006), is the pressure and tension on the status quo – a disruption of the family steady state. Family theorists argue that there are several key transitions that affect all families across their lifespan, for example, the transition to parenting after the birth of a child or the death of an elder, which are referred to as normative stressors. Normative stressors would rarely lead to crisis because most families are able to adjust and adapt to these changes and are generally considered as predictable. However, in addition to these normative events, there are a wide range of unexpected or non-normative stressors families experience in their lifespan, for example, from outside the family such as unemployment or within the family such as acute illness, trauma or an exacerbation of a chronic illness. These unexpected changes are highly stressful because they lack predictability. These changes or stressors, however, may be positive or negative in their impact on the family depending upon how the change or stressor is perceived. According to the family systems theory, both normative and non-normative stressors contribute to *morphogenesis* which is the ability of the family to develop and adapt to the changing needs of the family (see Chapter 2). It is important here to recognise that for some family carers, stress is not just seen as a negative effect on their mental health and well-being but also as playing a positive role in adaptation; psychologists refer to this as 'stress inoculation'. Meichenbaum's (2007) stress inoculation approach proposes that experience in dealing effectively with moderate-level stressors may inoculate individuals against the potentially pathogenic effects of subsequent stressful events. Progression into the maladaptive state conversely, due to a severe or prolonged stressor or multiple cumulative stressful insults, can have a deleterious effect (see Chapter 5). Distress is a term that is often used to describe this state. Whilst distress has many definitions, it is mostly characterised as a negative state in which coping and adaptation processes have failed to achieve homeostasis.

Crisis and Caregiving

A good starting point to understanding the term 'crisis' is to look at its origin. The word 'crisis' is derived from the Greek word *krisis* from *krinein*, which means 'to decide'. This definition emphasises the need for change in order to resolve a situation. Whilst family researchers introduced the term *crisis* for what is now called stressors in stress theory, the terms 'stress theory' and 'crisis theory' are often used interchangeably. We often hear family carers talking of being in a crisis or being stressed and both are universal and unique experiences but are fundamentally different.

Based on his work with families immigrating to Israel following World War II, Caplin (1964) provides a useful definition of crisis, stating that it occurs when individuals are confronted with problems that cannot be solved as individuals; people in a crisis are in psychological and emotional disequilibrium whereby their usual coping strategies fail to meet their needs. A crisis can be referred to as any intensive, rapidly changing, sudden or unexpected events that are beyond the individual's ability to respond to and achieve a homeostatic state. Boss (2002) makes a clear distinction between the terms 'stress' and 'crisis', viewing stress as a continuous variable experience, whereas crisis as either experienced by a person or not. It is worth noting that sometimes stress can be of catastrophic proportions, but not all stress is of this magnitude. Central to any definition of crisis is the notion that coping has failed, and most theorists seem to agree that the ensuing unstable state is temporary, although defining a time period for resolution is unclear.

In the event of a crisis such as sudden illness or trauma, carers' perceived inability to resolve these events or situations results in increased tensions, distress and a state of emotional unrest or instability, leading to an inability to cope or function (this can have adverse consequences; see Chapter 5). Several theorists have studied the crisis process, but Caplin (1964) was the first to describe the stages of a crisis reaction; other researchers have since based their ideas on Caplin's four distinct phases, which include the following:

1. In response to a situation/threat to a person's homeostasis state, an initial rise in tension occurs.
2. Persistence of the situation/threat increases the tension and disrupts daily living.
3. As tension increases, resolution of the situation may occur with new coping strategies, problem-solving responses and problem redefining.
4. If the situation continues, unresolved tension mounts and results in severe depression or psychological and social breakdown.

Perhaps you can resonate with these phases and have experienced them personally as well as in a professional capacity. In our experience, these phases manifest in interactions with families and relatives in different care contexts and in different behaviour guises. Understanding the underpinning theory can go some way to enabling our communication strategies, for example, but more of this is discussed in Chapter 6, where we explore interventions.

Although there appears to be no agreement in the literature as to the definition of stress, three broad theoretical perspectives have been extensively studied in the caregiving literature and offer a means of studying how caregivers adjust and adapt to stress. These include (1) stress as a response, i.e., physiological or biomedical models such as general adaptation syndrome (GAS) (Selye 1956); (2) stress as a stimulus psychosocial models, i.e., life events theory and the stress process; and (3) cognitive transactional process, i.e., transactional theory of stress (TTS) (Lazurus 1966). These three perspectives are discussed in the following sections.

Stress Models

Stress as a Response: General Adaptation Syndrome

The biological or physiological approach to stress, such as GAS, allostasis and allostatic load, suggests a direct cause and effect relationship and emphasises disease as a consequence. These approaches provide a conceptual basis for quantifying the physiological effects of the stress in carers. The characteristic set of physiological effects as a result of a stressor is referred to as the 'stress response'. The Hungarian endocrinologist Hans Selye was the first to define and measure stress adaptations in humans in the 1930s, and his seminal research remains influential today. Although the American physiologist Walter Cannon in the 1920s described the *fight-or-flight* response to perceived danger, it was Selye who argued that it was only the first stage in a series of reactions which he referred to as 'stress', a term he coined, and in his model of stress put forward a second stage called "resistance". Selye (1956) defined stress as

...a state manifested by a specific syndrome which consists of all the non-specifically induced changes within the biological system.

He called this biological response the GAS. For Selye, stress represents the effects of anything that seriously threatens our constant internal milieu or homeostasis. Selye also coined the term *stressor* to describe the agent that provokes the stress response. Stress, therefore, is the process by which the organism adapts to the stressor. The model assumes that regardless of a stressor, the same physiological response will occur and as a result, an adaptive response follows. During the second stage, *resistance*, the body focuses on physiological resources to manage the stressors (e.g. raised cortisol and adrenal levels); in other words, adaptation is sustained, but if these resources are exhausted, the body enters a final stage of exhaustion or cessation of the adaptation process during which the person is susceptible to disease and death. Although stress in Selye's model is perceived as negative, not all stress is unpleasant. Selye went on to introduce the term 'eustress' or positive stress, which can enhance functioning, giving over to positive feelings such as the 'feel good factor'. Eustress addresses the opportunity for personal growth and satisfaction for carers and helps to explain the more positive aspects of caregiving.

For Selye, all life events cause some stress. However, the GAS model says little about the person's prior experiences, perceptions or appraisal of stressors and pays limited attention to the influence of environmental or social contexts. Although any stressor or threat to the internal milieu of an individual is countered by the body's biological adoptive response, stress experienced by family caregivers cannot be viewed from this reductionist biological perspective alone. There needs to be an account of the interrelationships with other family members, i.e., the whole family unit together with psychological, social and environmental variables. Despite this criticism, as a basic model of stress, it remains useful.

Building on Selye's GAS, Sterling and Eyer (1988) described how individuals, when exposed to acute stress, seek physiological stability (or homeostasis) through an adaptive response known as 'allostasis'. The term 'allostasis' literally means *maintaining stability, or homeostasis, through change*, thus the body's biological cost of this adjustment to stress. The allostasis response describes the activation of nervous, endocrine and immune systems to meet demands of a stressor. In acute stress, the sympathetic–adrenal–medullary axis releases catecholamines such as epinephrine. In a longer-term stress response, the hypothalamic–pituitary–adrenal axis is activated and a consequential series of events then takes place, affecting many body systems, including the immune system, and enabling the body to respond to stress, thereby avoiding danger and increasing energy. This communication between the neuroendocrine and immune system constitutes a negative feedback loop which regulates responses to stressors and plays a major role in adaptation. However, long-term adjustment to the stressors (i.e. repeated and prolonged stressors such as those associated with caregiving) has negative consequences and is referred to as 'allostatic load'. In other words, allostatic load concerns the *wear and tear* on physiological systems as a result of repeated allostatic response (McEwen 1998). This allostatic load may result from multiple stressors, prolonged stress or an inadequate response to stress. It is argued that over time allostatic load affects various organs leading to an increased vulnerability to disease and infections (McEwen 1998, 2000), for example, elevated blood pressure during periods of perceived stress. We will return to this feature in Chapter 5. McEwen (2000), however, states that allostatic load is influenced by how an individual perceives stress, i.e., the brain controls the interpretation of events (threatening or non-threatening), and whether lifestyle behaviours such as diet and exercise can alter the stressor. Therefore, it must be noted that a family caregiver's perception of stress or self-reported stress is not necessarily equivalent to the stress measured by biomarkers such as cortisol levels.

Psychological Models of Stress and Adaptation: Stimulus-Based Theory of Stress

Life Events Theory

A focus on the entire family unit has formed the basis for family stress research since the 1930s and demonstrates the importance of family not only in creating stress but also in helping to manage it. Interest grew in the 1930s regarding the relationship between social, psychological and environmental factors and illnesses. In particular, Adolf Meyer influenced the development of connections between illness and stressful events and devised the life chart in order to chronologically document a person's major life events and significant illness experiences over a lifespan. Most notable among the other researchers progressing these ideas were Thomas Holmes and Richard Rahe, two psychiatrists who, in the 1960s, were among the first to systematically address the effects of changes in life circumstances on stress and who proposed a stimulus-based theory of stress entitled 'life events theory'. (Holmes and Rahe 1967). This theory proposed that changes that occurred as a result of major life events resulted in the body absorbing the psychological stress, and that, as a consequence, one's capacity to cope becomes reduced. Key points in this theory are that several life events increase a person's vulnerability to disease, illness and death and that any change which requires adaptation is stressful, which interestingly is consistent with Selye's approach. Since the 1970s, numerous studies on the relationship between life event stress and illness have used life events theory as a basis. Holmes and Rahe's research produced a weighting system for 43 critical life-changing events, called the social readjustment rating scale (SRRS), ranging from 100 (death of a spouse) to 11 (minor violation with the law); they argued that certain life events were predictive of stress-related illnesses. The SRRS, however, makes no mention of caregiving or caring for a family member but does rank a change in the health of a family member as 11 out of the 43 life events listed. Clearly this omission reflects the state of play during the 1970s whereby carers were largely invisible and unaccounted for in research endeavours.

It is now generally accepted that life events are a potent influence on mental and physical health. However, this SRRS theory assumes a uniform effect that can be measured by life event units and does not account for the subjective nature of life events, i.e., some life events may yield more stress than others and their meanings may vary from person to person. The SRRS index also does not inform us as to how, through time, the events may impact on a person's health.

In contrast to Holmes and Rahe's major life events of, Lazarus and Folkman (1984) proposed that a cumulative, relatively minor impact of stressors and pressures of everyday life can be a potent source of stress, arguing that these stressors can cause more suffering than major life events. These 'micro-stressors', such as frequent daily demands of caregiving which can be irritating, frustrating and distressing, are referred to as 'daily hassles'. Although daily hassles may seem of little consequence, during times of frequent and prolonged caregiving, e.g., hospital appointments, medication administration and daily chores, these daily hassles can adversely affect the caregiver's health. Moreover, whether they are unanticipated or anticipated, these daily hassles do mount up and contribute to major life stressors.

Researchers with an interest in the relationship between daily hassles and family stress have sought to develop measures to assess family members' experiences of their impact. The first measure was devised by Kanner et al. (1981) known as the 'hassles scale', which includes health and well-being of a family member. Later developments in measures ensued with the publication of the hassles and uplifts scale (Delongis et al. 1982, 1988), and the caregiving hassles and uplifts scale (Kinney and Stephens 1989) was developed for assessing daily stressors of caregivers of people with dementia. Rollins et al. (2002) refined an earlier version of the family daily hassles assessment instrument developed by Lee (1986) and devised a Family Daily Hassles Inventory in an attempt to measure the stress of day-to-day family life. They propose that this inventory offers three additional refinements: (1) a family focused assessment, (2) a shorter assessment, and (3) an assessment that takes into account all dimensions of daily hassles. Furthermore, they argue that this inventory focuses on the family as a unit and can provide a useful measurement of family stress. These scales and inventories highlight the perceived importance and severity of daily events in caregivers lives. According to Lazarus and colleagues, 'uplifts' or positive minor events that make you feel good serve a protective function acting as a buffer against stress. The impact of these daily hassles on family caregivers may be dependent upon several factors – frequency, intensity, number of competing hassles and any coexisting major life events. Some hassles may be easier to handle than others and this reiterates the point that not all carers can be viewed homogenously in their ability to adapt and cope with daily hassles of caregiving in the same way.

Thinking Box

Can you list some possible daily hassles a family caregiver experiences that you have had contact with?

How did you identify the hassles?

Did you have an opportunity to discuss their impact? And with whom?

Stress Process Model: Sociological Perspective

An important sociological model that has been extensively studied and applied is Pearlin's caregiver stress process model, initially published in 1981 as a conceptual model known as the *stress process*. Leonard Pearlin proposed that an individual's stress process is affected by a number of conceptual factors, namely source, mediators and outcomes of stress. Interestingly, Pearlin (1989) went on to state that four domains of the stress process are involved and these are

1. Background and context of stress (e.g. caregiver's age, race, socioeconomic status, gender and other demographic variables)
2. Stressors (primary stressors directly related to caregiving and secondary stressors to indirect factors such as social burden)
3. Mediators of stress (factors that lessen the effect of the stressor), which include coping strategies and availability of social support
4. Outcome of stress, i.e., changes in the physical and psychological well-being of the caregiver

Thus, according to Pearlin et al. (1990), the four domains of the caregiver stress process model interact with each other and determine the outcome. Pearlin and his colleagues argue that stressful life events and chronic life strains are part of everyday life and that the origins of stress emerge from society and may surface in the form of disruptive events or as a consequence of more persistent hardships and problems. In addition, they argue that exposure to one stressor may lead, over time, to exposure to other secondary stressors, a process called 'stress proliferation'. Stress proliferation in the context of caregiving can result from the strain of adopting the caregiving role which gives rise to struggles in family roles.

In addition, clusters of stressors, some of which may persist over time, can contribute to the *allostatic* load referred to earlier. In the caregiver stress process model, the outcomes of stress on caregivers may include disturbances in mood (e.g. depression or anxiety) or decline in physical health. We will discuss this in more detail in Chapter 5.

Of note, since its introduction, this model has undergone considerable refinement and several studies apply the model as a theoretical framework. Although this model originated for dementia, it has been applied in studies on caregivers of people in diverse populations.

Life Course

More recent approaches to stress have explored the effect of life events and chronic strain over time (i.e. as a person ages), which is referred to as 'life course' (Elder 2000), on stress and health behaviours. This perspective focuses on the longer view of how stress experiences may shape future outcomes and how this interplay may be different at varying points in a person's life course. The life course perspective in essence takes into account the individual lives and social change or life events over time. In a similar vein, Lazarus and Folkman (1984) identified that the significance of *life events* depends on the person's life history, life stage and circumstances, which leads to an individual experience with individual meaning. Caregiving can thus be viewed as a life course role that one enters and exits. This has significant implications for research about caregivers and understanding caregiving for two key reasons. First, assessing carers at any one point in time may only provide a 'snapshot' and does not capture differences as time progresses. Second, it highlights the importance of understanding the bigger picture of a carer's in-depth experience. A carer's previous experience of caregiving and life events will influence their caregiving behaviours and experiences.

We argue that taking a holistic view of family context, one that values a person's histrionics in terms of life course, rather than taking a snapshot of their experiences, may help to provide nurses with a more comprehensive view of a carer's experiences and needs. It is here that nurses need to be mindful of the carer's stress contexts to guide their assessments so as to identify stress factors that may not be obvious or that may not otherwise be considered important or relevant. However, a major criticism of these stress models is the lack of focus on the positive outcomes of caregiving. This dynamic relationship between carer and care recipient and positive experience and outcomes will be discussed in more detail in Chapter 5.

Psychological Stress (Transactional Theory of Stress)

Two key concepts critical to understanding psychological stress are the individual's cognitive appraisal or understanding of the situation and the individual's efforts to manage the situation, i.e., coping. Psychologist Richard Lazarus is one of the most influential researchers on stress and coping, and his stress theory is commonly adopted in caregiving research, so it is important that it be understood in order to fully appreciate carers' behaviours and responses to caregiving. One of the main factors affecting how the family copes is their personal perception and attitudes to the stressors, or, in other words, the evaluative or appraisal process which occurs in response to a stressor. This appraisal of a stressful situation is a central tenet of Lazarus's TTS and coping sometimes referred to as the cognitive relational approach. In this context, stressful experiences are understood as person–environment transactions.

Transactional theory of stress (TTS), or the appraisal theory of stress, was developed by Lazarus (1966) as a result of studies on peoples' stress levels. He observed that the way people think about stress had an impact on their stress levels. At the heart of this theory are two processes – appraisal and coping – and Lazarus emphasised individual appraisal of harmful threatening or challenging events and how this may impact their emotions and coping abilities. Over time, his theory was refined and developed to encompass the relationship between antecedent variables, mediating processes and outcomes and is explored in more detail in the book *Stress, Appraisal and Coping* (Lazarus and Folkman 1984), later revised by Folkman (1997) whereby she added the need to consider not just the negative emotions but also the role positive emotions have in the stress process. This appraisal process is based on the premise that individuals are constantly appraising their situation/environment and that a life event is not automatically a source of stress; rather, it is an individual's appraisal of stress that determines whether it is stressful or not.

Lazarus and Folkman (1984) conceptualised three types of cognitive appraisal: primary, secondary and reappraisal. When an individual is faced with a stressor, the cognitive appraisal or evaluation of the significance of what is happening is referred to as the primary appraisal, i.e., whether what is happening is personally relevant or significant. The situation or event can be appraised as being irrelevant (neutral), stressful, challenging or positive or threatening and harmful (negative). A secondary appraisal also occurs, at the same time as the primary appraisal, which involves the individual's evaluation of their available coping strategies and to what extent they can deal with the demands. Within this context, the level of stress experienced results from the amount of stressors 'out stripping' the resources to cope. Lazarus and Folkman (1984) suggested that an event will be perceived as stressful if a person believes that the stress will exceed their coping capability. If an event is seen to pose a threat or harm and if the concerned individual feels that they do not have the resources to cope, then negative psychological and physical effects may ensue, and this is explored in more detail in Chapter 5. This appraisal process is dynamic and changeable. As a carer evaluates the situation and gathers new information, a reappraisal of the situation may occur. This may intensify or attenuate the initial stress response. For example, a situation that was originally thought to be challenging or threatening may be reinterpreted as benign. Alternatively, a situation that was initially thought to be irrelevant or not stressful may later be appraised as stressful. In the context of caregiving, this has particular importance for two main reasons. First, it helps to explain the more positive experiences of caregiving as caregivers positively reappraise or reframe their situation; we will discuss this later in Chapter 5. Second, given that caregiving is a dynamic process and as a consequence of the changing circumstances and demands of their loved ones, a caregivers' stresses will undoubtedly change in significance over time. What was once thought to be stressful later, as their caregiving journey unfolds, blurs into insignificance as the reality of the magnitude of their situation is realised and new stressors are perceived as more stressful.

In some cases, the demands placed on a carer can either exceed or push them to the limits of their ability to cope. The notion that stress originates as a result of the interaction with the external environment and internal state of a person can help to explain why some caregivers are less affected by caregiving stress than others. One extreme example of the effect of the ongoing demands of caregiving was exemplified in a well-publicised case of Tracy Latimer, a 12-year-old Canadian with severe cerebral palsy, who was gassed by her father in 1993. In this case, Robert Latimer expressed his feeling of stress when caring for his daughter and the sense of helplessness regarding his child's future. He was charged with second-degree murder and sentenced to prison, which aroused considerable controversy in the press and caregiving literature.

To understand a caregiver's adaptations to their caregiving role, it is necessary to take into account the complex nature of this stress process and how this affects the caregiving experience. In Lazarus and Folkman's (1984) TTS, an individual carer's pattern of stress response can be reduced by changing their perception or appraisal of the potential threat. As individuals (carers) differ in their appraisal of their situation in the context of caregiving, nurses cannot assume that all family caregivers will perceive the situation the same way. Understanding that family members will appraise their stressors differently emphasises the importance of looking at all members of the family in the context of their unique caregiving situation and not treat them as a homogenous group. Essentially, if nurses treat all family caregivers alike, then support and interventions may fail or be ineffective.

Several variables that have been identified that could influence family members' perceptions and experiences of a stressful situation include carers' individual values, beliefs and commitments; personal characteristics (personality, motivation and intellect); society; gender; ethnicity; socioeconomic and marital status and stage of the family life cycle, i.e., structure and composition.

DeLongis et al. (1982) tested the impact of stress on health and mood and found that individuals with low self-esteem and unsupportive social relationships were more vulnerable to stress-related illnesses and mood disturbances than those with higher self-esteem and close social relationships.

Key Points

- Family caregiving has the potential to cause significant stress.
- Stress has been defined by many different disciplines and can be viewed from three main perspectives.
- Stress experience is individualistic and can be mediated by several factors.
- Stressors either begin or end in the family.

Family Stress Theory: Social Systems Perspective

Since Selye's GAS, the subject of individual stress has been studied for many years from several perspectives, including psychology, sociology, psychiatry and anthropology. We have explored stress theories to help understand caregivers' responses to the stressors of caregiving. From a family perspective, stress is underpinned by sociological social systems theory (discussed in Chapter 2), which permits exploration beyond the individual family member to the influences of wider social factors. The subject of family stress has developed relatively recently, beginning in the 1930s, with researchers such as the sociologist Robert C. Angell (1936), who studied how families coped with economic hardship during the Great Depression in America and observed that some coped better than others with the sudden loss of income. Angell concluded that families that were the most adaptable were called 'plastic families', referring to their flexibility in their family structure. He conceptualised that integration, which he defined as bonds of coherence and unity, and adaptability were key factors of a family's ability to cope with challenges. Interestingly, these two key factors formed the basis for the Olson et al. (1979) circumplex model of family systems (see Chapter 2).

After studying immigrants living in poor housing conditions, Earl Koos, another sociologist, proposed the term 'roller-coaster mode' (Koos 1946) in an attempt to provide the first framework of family stress emphasising the experiences and ways of coping with stress

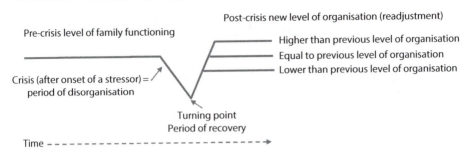

Figure 3.1 Roller-coaster model of family adjustment to crisis. (Adapted from Koos, E.L., *Families in Trouble*, King's Crown, Morningside Heights, NY, 1946; Hill, R., *Families under Stress*, Harper & Brothers, New York, 1949.)

over time, which he called the 'profile of trouble'. His framework proposed that the initial stressor or *trouble* causes a decrease in family organisation and interaction which varied in families, and this was followed by a recovery period, hence the roller-coaster analogy. Later, Reuben Hill, a social scientist working for the U.S. army, redefined the profile of trouble and renamed it the 'roller-coaster model of family adjustment to crisis'. This model describes four stages when faced with a crisis – crisis, a process of disorganisation, a period of recovery, during which the family may use a variety of coping strategies to rectify the situation, and a new level of organisation or readjustment which may be higher, equal or lower than before the onset of the stressor (see Figure 3.1).

Any disablement of a family member, for example, due to illness, trauma or diseases, inevitably involves the need for reorganisation of family life as depicted by the model (Figure 3.1). However, the model has been criticised over the years for several reasons – oversimplifying family stress, viewing stress as a linear process, failing to recognise that families may be subject to multiple complex stressors and there may be an accumulative effect and not taking into account that not all families can reorganise themselves. Despite this, the model does provide an understanding of how families adjust to crisis and acknowledges that a crisis does not occur in a vacuum. Perhaps, more importantly, it provides a basis for understanding family resilience, as the model identifies the ability of families returning or gaining a higher level of organisation than prior to the crisis, or, in other words, resiliency and thriving.

Hill (1949, 1958), whilst investigating the effect of war-induced separation and reunion on families, based on his earlier work and that of Angell and Koos, pioneered the development of family stress theory – the 'ABCX formula'. This linear theory, now better known as the ABCX model, forms the basis of most family stress models today, which earned him the status of 'father of family stress research' (Boss 2002). The ABCX model depicts the families' response to crisis as a roller-coaster ride with three key influencing factors that he denoted by the letters A, B and C. This model is shown in Figure 3.2.

Two complex variables in Hill's ABCX theory of family stress act to buffer the family from acute stressors – B resources and C perception of the stressors. According to this model, the lack of variables B and C would be a significant predictor of family crisis. In the C factor, the family's perceptions, meaning and appraisal of the stressor, reflects the family's values and

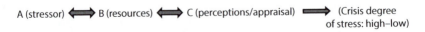

Figure 3.2 ABCX model of family crisis. (Adapted from Hill, R., *Social Casework*, 49, 139, 1958.)

beliefs along with their previous experience of dealing with stressors. According to Hill, families differ in their interactions between each other and the environment in which they live. Family adaptability or the X factor (crisis) can be understood as a continuous variable as a result of ABC, in other words, the amount of family disruption, disorganisation and inability to cope and restore stability that occurs. Thus, the interplay between variables A, B and C results in family stress. Boss (2006) argues that in a crisis (X), the family is temporarily immobilised and incapacitated and does not function properly. An important note in the family crisis model is the assumption that carers and family members can cope with disruption if there are sufficient resources (psychological and social) to meet the demands, in other words, the ability to select and utilise effective coping strategies.

In summary, family caregiving is often unplanned and unexpected and coupled with a lack of previous experience, which can increase the perception of stress; family caregivers are undoubtedly vulnerable to considerable stress. The cause of stress and the ways individuals and families adjust and adapt to stressors invariably differ considerably according to their caregiving situations. Some families may not have the required coping skills or an ability to develop or adapt to stressors. However, all families find resources either within the family or outside the family to help them cope with or manage stress in their lives. Although families vary in their ability to adapt, several factors have been identified that influence a family's ability to change and adapt and these include culture, education, gender, age and learning styles.

Clustering of Stressors: 'Pile-Up'

Because the demands and environment of carers and families change over time, rarely do families deal with one stressful event at any one point in time. In reality, what happens is that family crises evolve and are resolved over time alongside an accumulation of demands. Hill (1958) introduced the notion of *pile-up* to explain the complexity of families facing several expected (normative) and non-expected (non-normative) stressors simultaneously. Pile-up accounts for the fact that most families can accommodate demands and needs from all areas of family life, but when these stressors exceed a certain threshold, they are forced to reorganise. For family caregivers, this is particularly relevant, and as they embark on their caregiving responsibilities, they often experience several stressors at once – role changes, financial strain, changes to family life and restriction on personal freedom as they cope with their ill family member. This concept of stress pile-up is a notable consideration in supporting family caregivers crucially because a narrow focus on one stressor potentially overlooks the complexity of other stressors and their relationships with each other. These cumulative stressors may affect a carer's ability to adapt and adjust to their carer's role, and according to Boss (2006), pile-up of stressors can overwhelm family systems. Hill's notion of pile-up resonates with cumulative impact of minor daily hassles associated with caregiving, as discussed earlier.

Double ABCX Model

The 1970s and 1980s saw a period of modifications, adaptations and expansions to the ABCX model. Most notable of these were by two family social scientists McCubbin and Patterson (1982, 1983b), who built on Hill's model of stress and introduced an additional variables, the 'double factor', into the model and produced the double ABCX model (Figure 3.3). These researchers wanted to take into account the effect of time in the process of adjustment and attempted to explain why some families are more able to adapt to crisis than others.

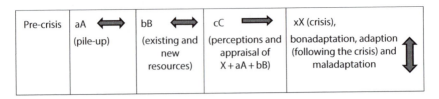

Figure 3.3 The double ABCX model. (Adapted from McCubbin, H.I. and Patterson, J.M., Family stress and adaptation to crises: A double ABCX model of family behavior, in Olson, D.H. and Miller, R.C., eds., *Family Studies Review Yearbook*, Vol. 1, Sage, Beverly Hills, CA, 1983a, pp. 87–106; McCubbin, H.I. and Patterson, J.M., The family stress process: The double ABCX model of family adjustment and adaptation, in McCubbin, H.I., Sussman, M. and Patterson, J.M., eds., *Social Stress and the Family: Advances and Developments in Family Stress Theory and Research*, Haworth, New York, 1983b, pp. 7–37.)

Based on surveys of wives of men who were either missing or were a prisoner of war during the Vietnam War, McCubbin and Patterson incorporated Hill's pile-up concept into the A of their double ABCX model (aA) explaining that several factors or stressors contribute to the pile-up in the family system, including hardships arising from stress, residual stress from previous events that may be exacerbated by new stress, normal transitions that occur in family life, family efforts to cope and ambiguity within the family. The bB factor, which represents the family adaptive resources, consisted of existing resources, including traits, characteristics or abilities of an individual family member or family system, and new *b* expanded resources which are generated in response to the stress, the most notable of which is the external resource of social support. When a family has sufficient and appropriate resources, they may perceive stressor events as manageable and therefore be less likely to perceive it as a challenge. Internal family resources such as family cohesion and adaptability have been suggested to be the most successful in adjusting to stress as in the circumplex model (see Chapter 2) (Olsen et al. 1980). Understanding that family resources act as buffers to moderate the effect of stressor events on family stress processes is an important consideration for nurses in supporting families and caregivers (we will return to this in Chapter 6 where we explore interventions to support family caregivers). The cC refers to the ability to reappraise and finally gives new meaning or understanding of the implications of stressors on self, relationships with others, priorities and future goals. Finally, the double xX refers to family crisis and adaptation and denotes family disorganisation and the need to adapt not only to a crisis but to a new level of family functioning.

Thinking Box

Identify the main stressors in a family that you have cared for. How did they react to these stressors?

How did they perceive such stressors/crisis?

How did this impact upon the family?

What do you think helped and what hindered them in dealing with the stressors?

In 1987, McCubbin and McCubbin expanded on the double ABCX model to develop the typology double ABCX model, now referred to as the FAAR (McCubbin and McCubbin 1987). These models reflected the change in focus from causes of stress and family weaknesses to concentrating on family strengths and the growing interest in resilience in stress theory. Although researchers and theorists have added to the original ABCX model, the basic principles remain the same, and considerable research over the past few decades has supported its application in a variety of contexts.

Key Points

- The ABCX and the double ABCX provide a framework to understand family stress.
- Stress results from the imbalance between resources capacity and the demands placed on the family.
- Family crisis can derail a family.
- How the family confronts and manages stressors along with buffers involved are critical to the adaptation of family members.

Resiliency

In conjunction with the development of the stress process, the construct of resilience also attracted growing attention in the 1970s and 1980s as a means of understanding why some individuals, despite their stresses, were able to positively adapt, and the researchers called this 'resilience'. Resiliency literature originally emerged through research that explored young people living in poverty or abuse in the 1970s. British psychiatrist Michael Rutter's (1979) study of children with mentally ill parents revealed that these children developed positive outcomes and did not develop mental ill health. Similarly, based on several other seminal studies in the 1970s, which focused on children in various conditions such as living with schizophrenic mothers, maltreatment and chronic illness, research began to reveal children's ability to adapt and thrive in these adverse conditions (Garmezy 1970, 1971, 1974; Werner and Smith 1982). These children were described as having extraordinary strength and inner resilience. This research began to overturn the negative assumptions about children growing up in severe adversity (hardship or suffering associated with difficult events or circumstances) and began to form the argument that many factors can help an individual thrive in adversity. Later years saw the focus of research on these underlying factors and processes in resilience, and it has since been expanded in many fields of research, including caregiving. This growing interest stemmed from both the desire to understand the risk and protective factors and how this information might be applied clinically, i.e., to support interventions. This evolving research saw a shift in emphasis from the negative stress process to a more positive emphasis on the strengths and capacities of individuals when under stress. However, typically, families have some internal strengths that they use for managing stress in their family system which is often referred to as resilience or a strong sense of coherence.

Resilience Defined

Despite the growing literature and research over that past 40 years in resilience, there appears to be no consensual single definition. The term 'resilience' has itself been defined and viewed in a range of ways – a trait, a process and an outcome. A useful starting point is offered by its Latin origins *resilire*, which means to recoil or leap back. Rooted in physics, the term refers to metals that were able to recoil or spring back into shape after bending. Boss (2006) indeed refers back to this original notion and describes it as the individual's ability to stretch or bend in response to stressors and strains in life, including challenging events such as trauma and illness. Norman Garmezy, one of the most important pioneers in the study of resilience, argues that resilience had to be viewed as a process and not as a fixed attribute of an individual. Similarly, Rutter (1993) contends that resiliency is a process, arguing that it is the capacity for successful adaptation in adversity and the ability to bounce back after encountering difficulties, negative events or tough times. Cameron et al. (2007) adds that the process of resilience is scaffolded by environmental, cultural and social psychological and physiological processes. Patterson (1995) regards resilience as one aspect of family functioning, i.e., as an ability to maintain a balance between change and stability within the family. Masten (2001) later stated that resilience is a basic human adaptive system and comes from *ordinary magic*, emphasising the common, normative human resources that she argues are present in all individual and families. Resilience can be defined as 'the capacity of a dynamic system to withstand or recover from significant threats to its stability, viability or development' (Masten 2011, 494). Put simply, resilience is the act of surviving despite stressful circumstances (Bonanno 2004). Boss cautions about the term 'resilience', stating that whilst it may refer to adaptability that Hill (1949) found to be present in those families who were able to withstand stress, it may not always be good to cope or be resilient. For example, it may be better for a caregiver to admit that they are unable to cope rather than trying to carry on. By letting go, facing the crisis and seeking help, a change and reorganisation of the family can occur. This may result in appropriate social support being instigated and the family needs being better met.

Despite myriad definitions of resilience, common to most are two key concepts: overcoming adversity and positive adaptation. Also, what seems to be common amongst the researchers is the belief that it is the engagement with stressful or adverse condition that makes a family resilient, not the avoidance of the conditions. In summary, resilience is a complex disposition and has been the subject of a number of studies and involves more than surviving a crisis but offers the potential for individual and family growth. The ability to revoke and endure the uncertainty and distress of a caregiver, which is referred to as resilience, is both individual and a family phenomenon. What appears to be critical is that resilience can only develop during times of adversity not despite it. The view that resilience is not a static process and can be affected by developmental changes raises several important points in relation to caregiving: that all carers possess the potential for resilience and that resilience has the potential to change over the life course of a carer. Also what seems to be critical in determining an individual's level of resilience is the interaction between the carer and the broader environment and their individual perceptions. This validates and highlights the importance of the transactional relationship between the individual caregiver and the environment, as highlighted in the transactional stress process (Lazarus 1966), and reemphasises the notion that viewing stress as an isolating event that evokes a response is insufficient in explaining the varying responses to stress.

Thriving, Surviving and Recovery

In general, we have seen that resilience is the ability to successfully adjust to adversity and maintain an equilibrium; however, the concept of thriving is also associated with positive adaptation. Thriving, which literally means to flourish or grow, represents either gain or benefit from a stressful event. These gains may include the acquisition of new skills and knowledge, confidence, strengthened personal relationships and mastery (Carver 1998). In the context of caregiving, any gain that enhances a caregiver's individual functioning or well-being thus meets the criterion of thriving. This notion that the person is able to thrive and grow from adversity has more recently been added to the multidimensional construct of resilience and represents a kind of growth. Indeed, Boss (2006) states that resilience is more than coping and overcoming, but also about thriving under adverse conditions. Similarly, Bonanno (2004) describes resilience as the ability to bounce back to the level of functioning equal or greater than before the crisis. Carver (1998), however, makes a clear distinction between thriving and resilience, noting that the former should be 'reserved to denote the homeostatic return to a prior condition', whilst thriving denotes 'the better off afterwards experience' (p. 247). Thriving is an important concept as it helps to explain anomalies in family caregiver's outcomes; for example, following a crisis, a carer somehow seems to thrive. Whilst the term 'thriving' is not generally used in caregiving literature, some researchers have focused on the positive development or becoming stronger in difficult and uncertain times or positively adapting to significant adversity using inventories such as the post-traumatic growth inventory (Tedeschi and Calhoun 1996). We will return to this in Chapter 5 when we explore in more detail the positive aspects of caregiving.

In this context, surviving is the ability to achieve stability in mental and physical health and cope with stressors. In response, carers tend to adopt the term 'surviving', but in essence, we suggest that what carers are inferring is that they have resilience. Recovery and resilience, however, are two different entities or trajectories. Recovery refers to a trajectory in which an individual's normal functioning is temporarily halted, but then, after a period of time, is returned to the pre-event functioning, for example, when recovering from an injury. Whilst resilience is the individual's ability to maintain a stable equilibrium, there is no loss of function (Bonanno 2004). Another distinction worth noting is that resilience is different from coping, although it is often used interchangeably in the literature. Whereas resilience refers to the appraisal of the events or stressors, coping refers to the psychological and behavioural mechanism (strategies) employed following the appraisal of the stress which fosters adaptation. We will explore coping in more detail in Chapter 4.

Thinking Box

What characteristics distinguish those who are able to thrive from those who do not and what resources help and promote thriving?

What role can a nurse play in this process?

Risk and Protective Factors for Resilience

Given that some family members and carers are more resilient than others, it is important that nurses understand what risks and protective factors influence resilience. In an effort to identify and understand the influencing factors that may predict resiliency, some researchers have focused on the internal characteristics of the person. Others have explored contextual factors such as culture, the collective network of the family and the community recognising that resilience is not only a personal ability but also a result of a combination of factors. Rutter (1987) conceptualised two key factors – vulnerability and protective factors – as being opposite ends of a continuum; he viewed *vulnerability factors* as an individual's particular reaction to negative situations and perceived these to lead to maladjustment, and *protective factors* were identified as ameliorating or moderating the exposure to risk. He also perceived these mechanisms to be more concerned with *key turning points* in the lives of resilient individuals rather than *long-standing attributes* or given experiences, although these terms add confusion to the literature on resilience as they are used inconsistently and variably. Garmezy (1991) provides a triadic model of resilience which has been widely cited and helps to understand this process. This triad model describes the dynamic interactions amongst risk and protective factors on three levels: family, individual and the environment. It is beyond the scope of this book to explore risk and protective factors in any detail, but some key factors are evident from the literature that are noteworthy; these include the following:

1. Risk or vulnerability factors (any influence that negatively affects a problem)
   a. Interpersonal factors such as negative self-belief or confidence, difficulty in asking for help and perceived conflict between beliefs and practices
   b. Lack of caring and supportive family and/or environment
2. Protective factors (buffer, protect or prevent risk)
   a. Interpersonal or intrinsic factors such as cognitive factors, competences (e.g. problem-solving skills), optimism, motivation, self-belief and strong sense of self
   b. Stress appraisal and coping strategies
   c. Socioecological or extrinsic factors such as the presence of supportive relationships and perceived social support and resources and cultural factors (e.g. cultural traditions, religious rituals and ceremonies)

What seems to be important is that there are risks and protective factors which are not static or separate entities but are elastic and changing in nature. For example, what might be protective today for a family caregiver may become a risk factor tomorrow (and vice versa).

A decisive factor in developing resilience is how an individual perceives and processes an experience. Polk (1997) provides a useful four-dimensional construct of resilience based on a concept synthesis of the literature, which relates to the person's overall health and ability to return to the original or near-original position after the stressful situation, and this includes the following:

1. *Depositional pattern*: Physical and psychosocial attributes that contribute to the manifestation of resilience, including intelligence, sense of mastery, positive self-esteem and sense of self-confidence
2. *Relational pattern*: The intrinsic and extrinsic characteristics of relationships such as seeking close support from others and using social networks
3. *Situational pattern*: Cognitive appraisal skills and problem-solving abilities
4. *Philosophical pattern*: Personal beliefs such as positive perception of self and finding positive meaning from experiences

As we have highlighted, many factors intervene in the promotion of resilience, and one way of practically visually synthesising and understanding these factors together can be found in the casita model devised by two Belgian theorists Stefan Vanistendael and Jacques Lecomte (2000) whilst working in community development in Chile; see Figure 3.4. This model utilises the image of a Spanish house, casita (a small house), where each room represents a major potential factor for resilience and an area for development and interventions. Within the casita's foundation is the fundamental acceptance of the person for who they are, which emphasises friendship, connectedness and networks in resiliency. This is a reminder to nurses working with family caregivers to be non-judgemental and open to the situation of the family caregiver and to try to understand family caregivers as individuals. The attic represents opportunities for other experiences to be discovered

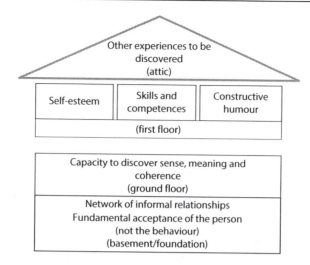

Figure 3.4 The casita model or house of resilience. (Adapted from Vanistendael, S. and Lecomte, J., *Le bonheur est toujours possible, Construire la résilience*, Bayard, Paris, France, 2000.)

and influence the process, representing hope. Fostering realistic hope is an important component of nursing practice, and nurses can play a pivotal role in promoting hope in family caregivers, which may help to equip them in dealing with the challenges of caring. This is explored in more detail in Chapters 5 and 6. The casita house is also a symbol of family relationships and a place of safety and warmth, all of which are important aspects of family life and connectedness. The model is simple, non-hierarchical and symbolically may help nurses to focus on the varying factors influencing resilience in their work with family caregivers. Further, the holistic nature of the model resonates with the principles of holistic nursing care, i.e., caring, relationships and interconnectedness. The casita also makes links with spirituality and finding meaning as understood by Viktor Frankl and sense of coherence which resonates with salutogenesis (Antonovsky 1987), both of which are explored in more detail in Chapter 4.

Family Resilience

In addition to seeing individual family members as potential resources of resilience, the family as a whole is of growing interest. Family resilience refers to families confronting together and managing stresses and challenges and how they adapt together to changes. Like individual resilience, not all families continue to live together and respond positively to challenges that ill health and injury create; some do not cope well at all and break up. The positive reaction to stressors has been described as family resilience, and like an individual's resilience, family resilience is an ongoing process. Its origins lie in the study of individual resilience, and it is an emerging concept. Whilst individual resilience is rooted in psychology and pathology as discussed earlier, the term 'family resilience' has relatively recently been used and has its roots in family stress management and prevention (McCubbin and McCubbin 1993; Walsh 1998). The premise being that adversity, whatever that may be, impacts the whole family. Walsh crucially views family resilience as a flexible construct that encompasses different family strengths in different contexts and at different points in the family life cycle. Hawley and DeHaan (1996, p. 293) provide a seminal definition of family resilience:

> ...the path a family follows as it adapts and prospers in the face of stress, both in the present and over time. Resilient families respond positively to these conditions in unique ways, depending on the context, developmental level, the interactive combination of risk and protective factors, and the family's shared outlook.

Thus, each family follows a unique trajectory to address risk which results in varying levels of adaptation. Perhaps more simply, family therapist Fiona Walsh defines family resilience as the coping and adaptation process a family faces as a functional unit (Walsh 2006). Walsh (2003) goes on to suggest a family resilience framework to guide prevention and intervention and so strengthen vulnerable families in crisis. Her framework, drawn from findings from numerous studies, outlines nine key processes for resilience within three domains of family functioning: family belief systems (making meaning of adversity, positive outlook, transcendence and spirituality), organisation patterns (connectedness, flexibility and mobilisation of social resources) and communication processes (clarity, open emotional sharing, collaborative problem-solving) (Walsh 1998). It is beyond the scope of this book to explore all of these domains in any detail, but all three are critical in the process of supporting family members in their caregiving roles.

Resiliency Model of Family Stress, Adjustment and Adaptation (FAAR) Model

Several researchers have added to the theories and models described throughout this chapter, which have helped our understanding of family resilience and, subsequently, caregiving. The most notable of them are McCubbin and McCubbin, who considered resilience as an important factor in family stress theory and expanded on their typology model of family adjustment and adaptation to develop their resilience model of family stress, adjustment and adaption (FAAR) (McCubbin and McCubbin 1991). This model has undergone several revisions since its original publication in 1991. In essence, the FAAR model emphasises the post-crisis adaptation phase in an attempt to explain the resiliency of some families and includes family type and family schema as salient factors in determining a family's level of adaptation to stressors. Family types include resilient family, who have a high degree of bonding and flexibility, and family schema is described as a family's beliefs and values, world view and ascribed meaning they give to a situation. Principally, these can be seen as an extension of the C factor (appraisal) in the ABCX and double ABCX models. Resilience in this model comprises two distinguishable but related family processes – adjustment and adaptation – in which a family draws upon recovery factors to promote an ability to *bounce back* and adapt in situations of family crisis (McCubbin et al. 1997). The FAAR model posits that family functioning is at optimal performance when there is equilibrium or balance between demands and capabilities.

Since the FAAR model, other researchers have refined family resilience terminology and proposed the family resilience model (Henry et al. 2015). These researchers identify four main elements of family resilience: (1) the presence of family risk, (2) family protection that facilitates families' abilities to restore balance between demands and capabilities after risk and which may protect against future risks, (3) family vulnerability that heightens potential for significant risk or a pile-up for risks and (4) short-term adjustment and long-term adaptation.

The concept of resilience plays a crucial role in understanding how families perceive and manage stress associated with family caregiving. Since the initial resilience research, a raft of research has advanced our understanding of resilience in relation to caregiving in several ways – understanding the processes that might account for resiliency or vulnerability can help to target intervention strategies, the identification of certain variables that promote or hinder resiliency in caregivers can help to understand resilience in a more holistic context and the development of resilience models and theories has helped our understanding of multidimensional constructs. Furthermore, resilience is a useful concept in stress processes and can enhance our understanding of and capacity to positively support families and caregivers. Each family caregiver's unique life circumstances along with their internal characteristics are central to their resiliency. Rather like a rubber ball that bounces back, caregiver and families have the ability to be resilient, although this may vary over their lifespan. Hence, all families have the potential to maintain their equilibrium despite significant adversity and as they become more resourceful, risks and vulnerabilities are reduced. Family resilience approach focuses on the strength and capacities of families and recognises the resourcefulness of families in adapting and providing care. From a family systems theory perspective, the more capable a family is to change internally in response to stressors, the better the family will be in adapting to new circumstances (Olsen et al. 1989).

By understanding the concept of resilience, nurses can help to identify carers who are able to overcome stressors and also understand the differences in how carers react in times of stress. Nurses can strengthen carer's resilience by recognising their challenges, supporting them through their caregiving journey and mobilising untapped resources so as to enable families to cope more effectively. Families often serve as an important protective factor for resilient individuals, but, equally, they may actually be a risk factor.

Key Points

- Stress, despite its negative connotations, eventually leads to adaptation and offers potential for growth.
- Resilience, in essence, refers to the ability to withstand or recover from adverse events.
- Resilience is a developmental process and can be learnt.
- Resilience is a multidimensional phenomenon that fluctuates as changes occur during carers' life course.
- Both protective and risk factors influence carers' level of resilience.

Chapter Summary

Caregiving is a complex process and many factors influence how the caregiver adapts to the stresses of caregiving. This chapter has provided a brief summary of some of the key theories related to stress, including their relevance to caregiving and potential to measure effects. The purpose of this chapter was to outline some of the key models related to stress in an attempt to help understand the adaptation and adjustment process in caregivers. Stress can be viewed individually or from a family perspective; the family stress response is dominated by the social system model such as the double ABCX and later the FAAR model. From the outset, we discussed adjusting and adapting in some detail to the process of change as a family responds to stress or crisis. Resilience, a more recent focus for caregiving research, refers to both the individual's and family's ability to cope with adversity and successfully deal with stress. Resilience is one of the constructs that protects or reduces vulnerability to stressors. We feel that the construct of resilience acknowledges that not all people struggle with negative events in their life such as acute trauma or illness. In the event of acute illness, trauma or disability, some family members achieve new insights and develop new abilities and grow from their experience of the adversity, so that in the future they are prepared to meet new crises with improved resources. However, not all families emerge from experiences of caregiving unscathed; many experience deleterious consequences and some undergo significant struggles in their efforts to cope. This is explored further in Chapter 5.

References

Aneshensel CS, Pearlin LI, Mullan JT, Zarit SH and Whitlatch CJ. (1995) *Profiles in Caregiving: The Unexpected Career.* San Diego, CA: Academic Press, Inc.

Angell RD. (1936) *The Family Encounters the Depression.* New York: Charles Scribner.

Antonovsky A. (1987) *Unravelling the Mystery of Health: How People Manage Stress and Stay Well.* San Francisco, CA: Jossey-Boss.

Bonanno GA. (2004) Loss trauma and human resilience: Have we underestimated the human capacity to thrive under extreme aversive events? *American Psychologist* 59(1): 20–28.

Boss P. (2002) *Family Stress Management: A Contextual Approach*, 2nd ed. Thousand Oaks, CA: Sage Publications, Inc.

Boss P. (2006) *Loss Trauma and Resilience.* New York: W.W. Norton & Company.

Cameron CA, Ungar M and Liebenberg L. (2007) Cultural understanding of resilience: Roots for wings in the development of affective resources for resilience. *Child and Adolescent Psychiatric Clinics of North America* 16(2): 285–301.

Caplin G. (1964) *Principles of Preventative Psychology.* New York: Basic Books.

Carver CS. (1998) Resilience and thriving: Issues, models and linkages. *Journal of Social Issues* 54(2): 245–266.

DeLongis A, Coyne JC, Dakof G, Folkman S and Lazarus RS. (1982) Relationship of daily hassles uplifts and major life events to health status. *Health Psychology* 1: 119–136.

DeLongis A, Folkman S, and Lazarus RS. (1988) The impact of daily stress on health and mood: Psychological and social resources as mediators. *Journal of Personality and Social Psychology* 54(3): 486–498.

Elder GH Jr. (2000) The life course. In E.F. Borgatta and Rhonda J.V. Montgomery (Eds.), *Encyclopedia of Sociology* (Volume 3), Second Edition. New York: Macmillan, pp. 1614–1622.

Folkman S (1997) Positive psychological states and coping with severe stress. Social Science and Medicine 45(8): 1207–1221.

Garmezy N. (1970) Process and reactive schizophrenia: Some conceptions and issues. *Schizophrenia Bulletin* 2: 30–74.

Garmezy N. (1971) Vulnerability research and the issue of primary prevention. *American Journal of Orthopsychiatry* 41(1): 101–116.

Garmezy N. (1974) The study of competence in children at risk for severe psychopathology. In: E. J. Anthony and C. Koupernik (Eds.) *The Child in His Family: Children at Psychiatric Risk: III*. New York: Wiley, p. 547.

Garmezy N. (1991) Resiliency and vulnerability to adverse developmental outcomes associated with poverty. *American Behavioral Scientist* 34: 416–430.

Hawley DR and DeHaan L. (1996) Toward a definition of family resilience: Integrating life-span and family perspectives. *Family Process* 35: 283–298.

Henry CS, Morris AS and Harris AW. (2015) Family resilience: Moving into the third wave. *Family Process* 64(1): 22–43.

Hill R. (1949) *Families under Stress*. New York: Harper & Brothers.

Hill R. (1958) Social stress and the family: 1. Generic features of families under stress. *Social Casework* 49: 139–150.

Holmes TH and Rahe RH. (1967) The social readjustment rating scale. *Journal of Psychosomatic Research* 11(2): 213–218.

Kanner AD, Coyne JC, Schaefer C and Lazarus RS. (1981) Comparison of two modes of stress measurement: Daily hassles and uplifts versus major life events. *Journal of Behavioral Medicine* 4(1): 1–39.

Kenney JM and Stephens MAP. (1989) Hassles and uplifts of giving care to a family member with dementia. *Psychology and Aging* 4(4): 402–408.

Koos EL. (1946) *Families in Trouble*. Morningside Heights, NY: King's Crown.

Lazarus RS. (1966) *Psychological Stress and the Coping Process*. New York: McGraw-Hill.

Lazarus RS and Folkman S. (1984) *Stress Appraisal and Coping*. New York: Springer.

Lee JL. (1986) Influences of daily routine on stress pile-up and families. Unpublished Masters Thesis, Iowa State University, Ames, Iowa.

Masten AS. (2001) Ordinary magic: Resilience processes in development. *American Psychologist* 56(3): 227–238.

Masten AS. (2011) Resilience in children threatened by extreme adversity: Frameworks for research, practice, and translational synergy. *Development and Psychopathology* 23(2): 493–506.

McCubbin HI and Patterson JM. (1982) Family adaptation to crises. In: H. I. McCubbin, A. Cauble and J. Patterson (Eds.) *Family Stress, Coping, and Social Support*. Springfield, IL: Charles C. Thomas, pp. 26–47.

McCubbin MA and McCubbin HI. (1987) Family stress theory and assessment: The T-double ABCX Model of family adjustment and adaptation. In: H. I. McCubbin and A. Thompson (Eds.) *Family Assessment Inventories for Research and Practice*. Madison, WI: University of Wisconsin, pp. 3–32.

McCubbin MA and McCubbin HI. (1993) Family coping with health crisis: The resiliency model of family stress, adjustment and adaptation. In: C. Danielson, B. Hamel-Bissell and P. Winstead-Fry (Eds.) *Families Heath and Illness*. New York: Mosby, pp. 21–63.

McCubbin HI and Patterson JM. (1983a). Family stress and adaptation to crises: A Double ABCX Model of family behavior. In: D. H. Olson and R. C. Miller (Eds.) *Family Studies Review Yearbook*, Vol. 1. Beverly Hills, CA: Sage, pp. 87–106.

McCubbin HI and Patterson JM. (1983b) The family stress process: The Double ABCX Model of family adjustment and adaptation. In: H. I. McCubbin, M. Sussman and J. M. Patterson (Eds.) *Social Stress and the Family: Advances and Developments in Family Stress Theory and Research*. New York: Haworth, pp. 7–37.

McCubbin MA and McCubbin HI. (1991) Family stress theory and assessment: The Resiliency Model of Family Stress, Adjustment and Adaptation In: HI McCubbin and AL Thompson (Eds.), *Families Assessment Inventories for Research and Practice*. Madison, WI: University of Wisconsin, Madison, pp. 3–32.

McCubbin MA and McCubbin HI. (1996) Resiliency in families: A conceptual model of family adjustment and adaptation in response to stress and crises In: H.I. McCubbin, A.I. Thompson, M.A. McCubbin (Eds.), *Family Assessment: Resiliency, Coping and Adaptation: Inventories for Research and Practice*. Madison, WI: University of Wisconsin, Madison, pp. 1–64.

McCubbin HI, McCubbin MA, Thompson AI, Han SY and Allen CT. (1997) Families under stress: What makes them resilient? *Journal of Family and Consumer Sciences* 89(3): 2–11.

McEwen BS. (1998) Protective and damaging effects of stress mediators. *New England Journal of Medicine* 338(3): 171–179.

McEwen BS. (2000) Allostasis and allostatic load: Implications for neuropsychopharmacology. *Neuropsychopharmacology* 22: 108–124.

Meichenbaum D. (2007) Stress inoculation training: A preventative and treatment approach. In: P. M. Lehrer, R. L. Woolfolk and W. E. Sime (Eds.) *Principles and Practice of Stress Management*. New York: Guilford Press, pp. 497–518.

Olson DH, Candyce SR and Sprenkle DH. (Eds.) (1989) *Circumplex Model: Systemic Assessment and Treatment of Families*. New York: Haworth Press.

Olson DH, Russell CS and Sprenkle DH. (1980) Circumplex model of marital and family systems II: Empirical studies and clinical intervention. *Advances in Family Intervention, Assessment and Theory* 1: 129–176.

Olson DH, Sprenkle DH and Russell CS. (1979) Circumplex model of marital and family systems: 1. Cohesion and adaptability dimensions, family types, and clinical application. *Family Process* 18(1): 3–27.

Patterson JM. (1995) Promoting resilience in families experiencing stress. *Pediatric Clinics of North America* 42(1): 47–63.

Pearlin LI. (1989) The sociological study of stress. *Journal of Health and Social Behaviour* 30: 241–256.

Pearlin LI, Mullan JT, Semple S and Skaff MM. (1990) Caregiving and the stress process: An overview of concepts and their measures. *The Gerontologist* 30(5): 583–594.

Polk LV. (1997) Toward a middle-range theory of resilience. *Advances in Nursing Science* 19: 1–13.

Rollins SZ, Garrison MEB, and Pierce SH. (2002) The Family Daily Hassles Inventory: A preliminary investigation of reliability and validity. *Family and Consumer Sciences Research Journal* 31(2): 135–154.

Rutter M. (1979) Protective factors in children's responses to stress and disadvantage. In: M. W. Kent and J. E. Rolf (Eds.) *Primary Prevention in Psychopathology: Social Competence in Children*, Vol. 8. Hanover, NH: University Press of New England, pp. 49–74.

Rutter M. (1987) Psychosocial resilience and protective mechanisms. *American Journal of Orthopsychiatry* 57(3): 316–331.

Rutter M. (1993) Resilience: Some conceptual considerations. *Journal of Adolescent Health* 14(8): 626–631, 690–696.

Selye H. (1956) *The Stress of Life*. New York: McGraw-Hill.

Selye H. (1976) *The Stress of Life*, Revised edition. New York: McGraw-Hill.

Sterling P and Eyer J. (1988) Allostasis: A new paradigm to explain arousal pathology. In: S. Fisher and J. Reason (Eds.) *Handbook of Life Stress, Cognition, and Health*. Chichester, UK: John Wiley & Sons, pp. 629–649.

Tedeschi RG and Calhoun LG. (1996) The Posttraumatic Growth Inventory: Measuring the positive legacy of trauma. *Journal of Traumatic Stress* 9(3): 455–471.

Walsh F. (1998) *Strengthening Family Resilience*. New York: Norton.

Walsh F. (2003) Family resilience: A framework for clinical practice. *Family Process* 42: 1–18.

Walsh F. (2006) *Strengthening Family Resilience*. New York: Guilford Publications.

Werner EE and Smith RS. (1982) *Vulnerable but Not Invincible: A Longitudinal Study of Resilient Children and Youth*. New York: R.R. Donnelley & Sons, Inc.

Vanistendael S and Lecomte J. (2000) *Le bonheur est toujours possible. Construire la résilience*. Paris, France: Bayard.

4

Coping Process and Coping Strategies

Introduction

The central mechanism through which family stressors, demands and strains are eliminated, managed or adapted is coping, and for this reason, this chapter explores in more detail the individual family and carer's ability to master, tolerate or reduce external and internal demands and conflicts as a result of caregiving. This chapter begins by exploring the concept of coping along with coping resources and coping strategies. The two dominant frequently cited categorisation of coping strategies, namely problem-focused and emotion-focused coping, are explored in more detail along with other coping strategies such as avoidance, distancing religious- and meaning-focused coping and humour. The chapter concludes with a discussion on the sense of coherence (SOC) as a means of explaining the variances in coping abilities of caregivers.

Caregiving can be challenging and stressful, as we have seen in the previous chapter, and the outcomes of stressful situations caregivers face can be largely dependent on their ability to handle or adjust and on the use of coping strategies. The literature proves that caregivers use different coping strategies to manage the difficulties they experience in their caregiving role. The mobilisation and the use of resources and coping strategies are crucial elements that impact on the stress experience and process. A number of factors are known to be related to effective coping strategies which need to be taken into account when addressing the coping process. It should be stressed from the outset that this chapter's discussion is not comprehensive, rather it provides an overview of some of the main coping strategies and the emerging research in the field. Understanding how different families cope can help nurses develop and implement successful effective intervention strategies.

Coping Defined

Coping is a fundamental, active and dynamic psychological process that we all perform to some degree on a regular basis. In general terms, it refers to the effort to ameliorate sources of stress and sustain a sense of psychological well-being. Several definitions have been offered over the years by theorists and researchers, and interest in coping grew in the main after the research on stress was published between 1950 and the late 1970s. Hans Selye introduced the notion of coping in his later work on stress, stating that coping can be defined as adapting to stress situations (see Chapter 3). Psychologists started studying coping back in the 1960s, and since then, research has significantly been influenced by the theoretical work of Lazarus and Folkman. Much of the research interest can be traced back to the work of Richard Lazarus in

1966 when he argued that stress consisted of three processes: primary appraisal, secondary appraisal and, finally, coping. Appraisal can be defined as an evaluative process that reflects the carer's subjective interpretation of an event or situation, and if it is perceived to be stressful, then stress occurs.

According to Lazarus and Folkman (1984), coping consists of cognitive and behavioural efforts to manage external or internal demands (and conflicts between them) that are appraised as taxing or exceeding the resources of the person. Mattsson (1972) defines coping as 'all the adaptational techniques used by an individual to master a psychological threat and its attendant negative feelings in order to allow him to achieve personal and social goals' (p. 805). The way a person interprets events is crucial because it shows whether he or she will cope with a situation successfully or become stressed by it (Antonovsky 1987). Others have suggested that coping refers to the personal management of a stressful situation that changes the meaning and reduces the threat (Pearlin et al. 1990). The emphasis seems to be on managing the requirements and difficulties caused by the stressful situation or event. Coping is characterised by both cognitive and behavioural efforts to manage internal and external pressures that may exceed the individual's current resources. Thus, coping is a means for achieving balance or maintaining the equilibrium. Simply put, coping refers to the way in which people attempt to relieve their stress (Endler and Parker 1990). Furthermore, it is a conscious, intentional and learned process representing what people do, not an outcome, and is considered effective if the stress is reduced.

Thinking Box

Does this resonate with you?

Can you think back to an occasion when you have had to cope with a stressful event, and what did you do?

Coping: Theoretical Perspectives

The literature indicates that coping can be viewed by two broad theoretical approaches – as a personality trait or style and as a process. Some theorists assume that differences in the use of coping strategies is linked to personality. The view that coping is a personality trait, which is the person's way or style of coping, is inherently stable and habitual, depending on how they view the world and themselves. The research into the role personality dispositions like self-esteem, locus of control and hardiness has in determining the degree to which a particular coping strategy is used remains unclear and inconclusive. However, there are some clear differences in the caregiving literature as to the use of particular strategies; we will return to this later in this chapter.

The process approach differs in that it views coping not as the person's disposition but rather as specific thoughts and behaviours in response to a stressful situation, and these may change over time. This process approach has been greatly influenced Lazarus and Folkman's (1984) transactional theory of stress. This theory argues that coping changes over time as the individual responds to the demands and appraisal and reappraisal of a stressful situation. The theory emphasises the interaction between stressors, individuals, their appraisal of a stressors and the efforts to manage the stress. Lazarus and Folkman's transactional model (1984) provides some basic principles in coping in that it emphasises a person's individual subjective appraisal of the situation. For further information on this model, see Chapter 3.

These varying definitions highlight that whilst there is general consensus of what constitutes coping, namely all efforts to manage a stressor, different researchers have placed emphasis on the varying aspects of the term. Central to the study of coping is both adaptation and adjustment, as we have seen in Chapter 3. People often examine and reexamine the outcome of a coping effort, which psychologists refer to as 'rumination'.

Maladaptive and Adaptive Coping

According to Folkman and Lazarus (1980), coping strategies serve two main functions: first to manage the person/environment relationship which is the source of stress and second to regulate stressful emotions. However, not all coping strategies have a positive outcome or are adaptive; some coping strategies can be negative or maladaptive. Adaptive coping is generally accepted to be constructive or positive coping leading to the re-establishment of a dynamic equilibrium that was disturbed by stress. Maladaptive strategies can be perceived as non-coping as the individual is unsuccessful in relieving their stress. Furthermore, maladaptive coping behaviours are generally thought to lead to a vicious circle which, by depleting the patient's resources, fails to stabilise the situation and aggravates the very problem it is supposed to solve and may affect the health and well-being of the individual. This is explored in more detail in Chapter 5. Another way of looking at these contrasting coping strategies is effective (adaptive) and non-effective (maladaptive) coping. Whether coping processes are considered adaptive or maladaptive depends on a number of important factors. These can be grouped into two main areas:

1. Situational factors, for example, the characteristics of the illness (severity and duration)
2. Personal factors, for example, personality and beliefs about the effectiveness of the coping resource

What may constitute as effective for one carer in a particular circumstance may not be so for another carer in similar circumstances. Thus, the effectiveness of coping is likely to vary according to the situation and the characteristics of the carer. Research indicates that people also use multiple strategies, often in combination, simultaneously trying to resolve the stress, but they may show a preference to certain strategies over others, for example, emotional or problem-solving coping. It is also important to understand that family carers may accept or adapt and cope at different points in time, and as the coping style of one family member changes, it impacts others in the family.

It is also important that nurses appreciate that a coping strategy that a carer may utilise to reduce the effects of stress can lead to both negative and positive outcomes. Therefore, coping strategies can help to determine whether the stress has a positive or negative effect on the individual. In addition, by being aware of the different coping strategies, nurses can help carers to avoid unnecessary additional stress by supporting effective coping attitudes of caregivers and intervene in order to change ineffective coping attitudes. Despite a carer's varying individual coping skills, as the stressors increase, so will the caregivers use of coping strategies. For example, deteriorating or changes to symptoms of a care recipient (e.g. progression of a disease) can result in a change in stressors and potentially increase caregiving demands and a consequential need to deploy more resources to cope. Furthermore, a strategy that initially was effective may then prove to be ineffective when the situation changes. For example, a carer may seek emotional support from her family during her spouse's acute illness, but once he is discharged home, the scenario will demand problem-solving strategies, i.e., the practicalities of managing her husband's needs. In the event of a crisis, i.e., a psychological and emotional disequilibrium, such as being confronted with the sudden illness of a family member, a family carer's normal coping strategies fail to meet their needs. Resolution of the crisis is very much dependent upon the carer's ability to utilise adaptive coping strategies. A key aim for nurses is to assist caregivers in regaining their pre-crisis equilibrium; however, in order to do this, a clear understanding of the carer's coping strategies is needed, which are discussed next.

Coping Styles and Strategies

Whilst coping defines the process of solving problems and situations, the mechanisms that individuals deploy are referred to as coping strategies or behaviours. Thus, coping strategies generally refer to specific behaviours or techniques that individuals deploy to manage a stressful situation. However, the literature also uses the term 'coping styles', often interchangeable with coping strategies, which can cause some confusion as it actually refers to a broader categorisation of coping behaviours.

Holahan et al. (1996) suggest that coping styles can be divided into active behaviour, active cognitive and avoidance behaviours. Active behavioural styles refer to external behaviours such as problem solving and seeking help; active cognitive styles refer to a number of internal processes such as acceptance, finding inner strength (meaning) and religious beliefs. Avoidance-focused behaviours include ignoring or avoiding and denial. Thus, these styles can be viewed in terms of how the individual responds to a stressor, internally (such as cognitive) or externally (behavioural).

Similar to these broad categories and frequently cited in the literature is the earlier work of psychologist Richard Lazarus, who, in 1966, identified two main forms of coping, which he termed direct action coping and palliative coping (intrapsychic). These were later renamed by Lazarus and Folkman (1984) as problem-focused coping (aims at modifying the sources of the problem) and emotion-focused coping (efforts to reduce the emotional effect of the stress), respectively. Building on the work of Lazarus, Moos and Billings (1982) offer a third category, appraisal-focused coping, which includes coping responses connected to logical analysis, cognitive redefinition and cognitive avoidance strategies. More recently, Folkman (1997) discovered that in stressful situations, people often seek out events that are meaningful or create positive meaningful experience out of ordinary, neutral life events. In light of this, Folkman revised her earlier stress process model (see Chapter 3) to include meaning-focused coping as a resource that is used when individuals face an unfavourable resolution or no resolution to a problem. Moreover, Folkman (2008) states that research studies support the distinction of meaning-based coping from other forms of coping. Meaning-focused coping includes strategies that involve creating, reinstating and reinforcing meaning in a stressful situation (Folkman 1997; Park and Folkman 1997). As Carver et al. (1989) argue, the distinction between problem-solving and emotion-solving coping, although important, is too simplistic. Nevertheless, the two main dimensions of coping problem-focused and emotion-focused coping remain consistent in the literature today. Several criticisms have been levied at this distinction, most notably that the categories are not clear or mutually exclusive, that there are many ways of coping which incorporate both dimensions and that there are other strategies that fall outside the two dimensions such as religious coping and humour. Besides, Pearlin and Schooler (1978, pp. 7–8) suggest 'coping, in sum, is certainly not a unidimensional behaviour. It functions at a number of levels and is attained by a plethora of behaviours, cognitions, and perceptions'.

Key Points

- Coping is a complex, dynamic, multidimensional development process.
- Coping is a conscious, intentional and learned process to reduce the effect of stress.
- Coping with stress can be adaptive (effective) or maladaptive (ineffective).

Problem-Focused and Emotion-Focused Coping

Problem-focused coping is sometimes referred to as instrumental coping; in principle it involves taking action to solve a problem. Endler and Parker (1990) used the term 'task-focused coping' instead. However, both include assessing the challenges or stressors and using problem solving and planning in an attempt to modify the source of stress, for example, the carer seeking information that is relevant to the situation and taking direct action to solve the problem. It may also involve social support for advice, assistance or information. These goal-directed strategies tend to be used when a carer feels that they can either change or have some control over the situation. Consequently, this may engender a perceived sense of control, purpose and meaning. However, for carers who usually deal with stress by using problem-solving coping when they face a new situation, such as the hospitalisation of their loved one, and information about the situation is not made readily available, it may create feelings of uncertainty and create unnecessary stress. Some researchers view problem-solving approaches as being the most useful strategy, and cognitive and emotionally focused efforts to be more likely to result in burnout, whereas problem-solving efforts such as confronting difficulties, seeking information and social support to be more effective (Almberg et al. 1997).

Problem-solving according to the social problem-solving model (D'Zurilla 1986) refers to problem-solving in the natural environment, where problems are defined as an imbalance between a demand and the availability of effective coping responses. Essentially, problem solving is a self-directed learning process that aims to work out or discover effective solutions to everyday problems and thus reducing or modifying the negative emotions that are associated with the problem. In this regards, it is an adaptive coping strategy. According to the social problem-solving model, individuals have an innate problem orientation which is either positively orientated leading to rational problem-solving skills or negatively orientated leading to ineffective problem-solving skills such as avoidance and an impulsive careless style. Caregivers who have a negative problem orientation are more likely to experience negative emotional as problem solving is impaired, thus interfering with the cognitive process of finding solution to the problem. Research clearly indicates that those caregivers who have a more negative problem orientation were more likely to report more depressive symptoms and less satisfaction with life than those who reported a more positive approach to managing problems in daily living.

Positive problem orientation involves the general belief that the carer can solve the problem (optimism); on the other hand, negative problem orientation tends to view problems as significant threat and questions their ability to solve the problem. In terms of the social problem-solving model (D'Zurilla 1986), a problem can also be perceived as a stressor when the problem becomes a significant challenge to an individual (see Chapter 3). However, unlike Lazarus' model of stress, which views problem solving as a form of problem-focused coping strategy, in the social problem-solving model, problem solving is viewed as a broader coping strategy encompassing both problem-focused and emotion-focused coping strategies. It is also worth noting that 'pile-up' of unresolved daily problems can lead to greater problems, as identified in Chapter 3.

Emotion-focused coping is a cognitive strategy that is more likely to be employed in situations when the individual can exert little control (Folkman and Lazarus 1980; Endler and Parker 1990). The aim of this coping strategy is to reduce negative emotions in response to adverse events or change the appraisal of the demanding situation or event. Examples of emotion-focused coping strategies may include reframing events and taking a positive point of view or seeking moral support, understanding and sympathy from other family members or friends (see Table 4.1). Emotion-focused strategies may also include using religion, humour or acceptance to lessen the effect of a stressor (Carver et al. 1989). By reappraising the situation, the carer may convince themselves that a problem is not worth worrying or stressing about. But seeking emotional support can be a double-edged sword: on the one hand, it can be adaptive, providing help to utilise problem-solving coping, and on the other hand, venting emotions may create more stress and thus be maladaptive. For example, using an emotion-focused strategy, such as expressing one's feelings, may actually have a negative effect of increasing a carer's negative emotions. However, when stressors are short-lived, emotion-focused coping may actually be adaptive, for example, in situations where a carer may not have much control.

Seeking information for some carers may help to relieve the stress associated with uncertainty or misconceptions that often occur in the caregiving role. Other writers, however, suggest that it is helpful to have a number of differing coping strategies that can be selected to address varying situations that the caregiver may face. For example, as Nolan et al. (1996) points out, problem-solving models are of little use if a certain problem cannot be solved. In such circumstances, looking at a problem from a different perspective is likely to be more helpful. However, in the case of dementia caregivers, Cooper et al. (2008) argue that although problem-solving strategies are useful, their effects may be less long-lasting when compared to the benefits of emotion-focused coping. Although problem-focused coping tends to be viewed as more adaptive, emotion-focused coping may be a better strategy when it is not possible to change the stressor or situation as often is the case in this caregiving role. On the contrary, emotionally focused coping, which often entails avoidance-oriented coping (e.g. denial), has been generally associated with general distress, more depression and the amplification of future problems. In general, it appears that emotion-focused strategies become maladaptive when used for long periods of time and when stressors are under the carer's control.

It is important for nurses not only to understand the differences between these two main categories but also to realise that they are not mutually exclusive and that carers often use both simultaneously. Furthermore, no single strategy is universally the most effective, but what seems to be key is the flexibility to deploy various coping styles according to a given situation.

Thinking Box

Think back to a family that you have recently been involved with; what coping strategies did they use?

Were those adaptive or maladaptive?

Table 4.1 Examples of contrasting coping strategies that families and caregivers may use

Active behavioural (problem-focused coping)	Active cognitive (emotion-focused coping)
Adaptive	**Adaptive**
• Seeking social support – developing a support group • Seeking advice and information in an attempt to understand and empower them with knowledge to determine how best to deal with the situation, for example, illness duration/course treatment pathways • Learning to become competent in their caregiving tasks • Identifying problems that can be solved and working through them • Redefining priorities and setting new goals that are aligned to the priorities • Liaising and working with nurses and other healthcare professionals • Identifying specific tasks that other family members or friends can do to help • Planning and evaluating solutions to the situation • Being suppressed to complete activities to focus on the situation • Restraining or holding back until an appropriate opportunity arises to take action, and not acting prematurely	• Seeking emotional support from others – venting or unburdening feelings, concerns and emotions to others, e.g., partner, friend • Normalisation (reducing the feeling of being different) • Seeking causes to the situation • Accepting support from other family members and friends • Positive reappraisal or reframing of the situation or problem • Acceptance • Cognitive reframing
Maladaptive	**Maladaptive**
• Trivialisation of issues • Rumination	• Clamming up and suppressing feelings • Clinging to the hope that the person will get better when this is unrealistic • Avoidance (withdrawing or avoiding others or situations) • Distraction and denial • Wishful thinking that the problems or issues will go away or a miracle will happen • Use of tobacco, alcohol and other substances; excessive spending and gambling to escape from the problem • Rumination (persistent and recurring negative thoughts that focus on the symptoms of distress and on its possible causes and consequences) • Self-blame

Sources: Carver, C.S. et al., *J. Pers. Soc. Psychol.*, 56(2), 267, 1989; Lazarus, R.S. and Folkman, S., *Stress Appraisal and Coping*, Springer, New York, 1984.

Key Points

- Problem-focused coping targets the stressor, whilst emotion-focused coping targets the person's emotional state.
- No single coping strategy is universally the most effective.

Avoidance and Denial Coping Strategy

Avoidance strategies such as denial, withdrawal and rumination are common strategies that family carers may engage in and essentially involve a strategy that protects a person from a threat. Endler and Parker (1990) note that an individual can use avoidance strategies by seeking out other people, i.e., social diversion or by engaging in substitute (distraction). This maladaptive approach to dealing with stress is often characterised by avoiding contact with people (e.g. family members or healthcare professionals), blocking out the situation, and may be detrimental to both carers and their loved ones. Avoidance coping in general involves the use of strategies that places the focus away from the source of the stress and the reaction to it. According to Lazarus and Folkman (1984), avoidance is an ineffective coping method that emotionally alienates the individual from the stress-related situation. Evidence suggests that in a variety of caregiver populations, a significant positive correlation is found between depression and the use of self-blame and denial as coping strategies (Bautista and Erwin 2013). Behaviours such as self-blame, venting, denial, avoidance or resignation have been associated with higher levels of emotional problems (Kim et al. 2007). In dementia caregivers, using avoidance coping strategies was found to be positively correlated with caregiver burden (Huang et al. 2015) and anxiety (Snyder et al. 2015). Avoidance and denial behaviours may even be harmful to a carer's health, for example, a spouse who denies help with her demented husband's needs may mean that she neglects her own physical health and well-being as she struggles on without help. In some carer groups, the use of avoidance has been found to be a common strategy. For example, Cotton et al. (2013) report that avoidance strategies such as denial, withdrawal and ruminations are common amongst carers of young people with psychosis. Whilst Onwumere et al. (2011) found that in carers of people with long-term psychosis, the use of avoidance strategy was associated with a greater level of carer distress.

Avoidant coping may be adaptive when a carer cannot change or control their situation. More specifically, carers may avoid, reject or postpone seeking information about their loved ones especially if they believe that it won't change their situation or feel that they have no control over their situation. Some carers may be motivated to seek information, when families are aware that information is missing, relevant and/or applicable, but some carers avoid seeking information. Thus, nurses should not assume that all carers are motivated to seek information about their loved ones; some carers may not want or avoid seeking information if it is of no value or if it becomes a hindrance. Equally, carers may seek information only if they perceive it to be of use or if it meets their needs. Case et al. (2005) argue that uncertainty may initiate and motivate carers to seek information to reduce their uncertainty, as typically uncertainty is associated with anxiety. In other words, family carers may make a choice to seek information. As the infamous American psychologist Abraham Maslow (1963) wrote, '…we can seek knowledge in order to reduce anxiety and we can avoid knowing in order to reduce anxiety' (p. 122). Maslow goes on to state that when we know fully and completely, then suitable actions follow automatically. It is important to appreciate that new information can both increase and decrease uncertainty depending on the situation, and this will vary according to previous experiences and other factors unique to the carer, such as their coping skills. However, research indicates that most family members prefer to be told the truth, even if it conflicts with their need for hope because 'not knowing' is worst (Fulbrook et al. 1999; Bond et al. 2003; Gaeeni et al. 2015).

Denial or refusing to believe that a problem or stressor exists can also be considered maladaptive especially if used over an extended period of time because the caregiver will have an inaccurate perception of reality. Also, attempting to stay away from the stressful event may mean, for some family members, that they isolate themselves from the rest of the family network. Denying that the situation does not exist or trying to act as if the stressor is not real will make the problem worse when they eventually face it.

Accepting and Distancing

Caregiving demands can be a tremendous drain on personal resources, but for some, they gain a balance in their lives through acceptance and distancing. Acceptance is recognised as a discrete coping strategy and can also be considered an element of both emotion-focused and problem-solving coping. Acceptance may also be considered the opposite of denial and implies that the carer has come to terms with the situation and realises that a given situation cannot be changed. Through acceptance, the carers acknowledge their situation and the reality of their loved one's condition or disability and that their caregiving role might be a long haul. Acceptance also means that they are able to set realistic expectations for both themselves and their loved ones. Distancing may involve not taking on responsibilities that others can do and letting go of what they are not able to change or influence.

Alternative Rewards Strategy

Moos and Billings (1982) identified a coping strategy that is undoubtedly familiar to all of us in times of stress, that of developing alternative rewards. This strategy involves trying to counter the losses involved in crisis by becoming involved in new activities and creating alternative sources of satisfaction. This strategy may manifest as both adaptive and maladaptive, in that adaptive alternative reward strategies include manual, intellectual or spiritual activities that keep the carer from pondering on the problem. However, maladaptive unhealthy behaviour, seeking alternative sources of satisfaction, may manifest itself by excessive smoking, alcohol consumption and substance misuse, which brings ill-health consequences.

Meaning-Focused Coping: Finding Meaning

One way that caregivers can positively appraise their caregiving experience is to find meaning. According to Reker et al. (1987), finding meaning involves making sense, order and coherence out of one's existence and plays an important role in the stress and coping process and in enhancing health and well-being. As caregiving is an innately helping role, aspects of caregiving that provide meaning are largely described as relating to caregivers' values and beliefs. Park and Folkman's (1997) model of coping makes explicit the role of beliefs and goals and the function of meaning in the coping process. The attributed meaning that people give to events is explicit in Lazarus and Folkman's transactional theory of stress (see Chapter 3), in that during primary appraisal, carers appraise stressful events according to their values and beliefs. Positive reappraisal, thus a form of meaning-focused coping, is the adaptive process by which stressful events are reconstrued as benign, valuable or beneficial. Similarly, within the stress process model (Pearlin et al. 1990), it is proposed that meaning is a mediator of stress. Although the word 'meaning' has many connotations, Park and Folkman (1997) refer to it as perceptions of significance, which involves an individual's ways of understanding. Creating positive appraisals and interpreting negative situations with a positive value/belief system lie at the core of meaning-based coping. In their model, Park and Folkman make a distinction between global meaning, which refers to an individual's beliefs and assumptions about the world, for example, religious beliefs and purpose in life, and situational meaning which refers to the meaning that is a result of the interaction between the person's beliefs and the appraisal of the interaction between the person and the environment. Situational meaning begins with the carer appraising the situation/event influenced by their own beliefs and values and followed by the search for meaning in the event. Similarly, Reker and Wong (1988) not only conceptualised meaning in this way but also offered a 3D existential construct of global meaning consisting of three mutually related components: cognitive, emotional and motivation.

In essence, Park and Folkman (1997) suggest that meaning-based coping is the management of the incongruence between global meaning and situational meaning. When this incongruence occurs as in sudden illness or trauma for family members, there is a need to search for meaning to achieve adaptation or a rebalance. During adaptive meaning-focused coping, a carer achieves either a change to their beliefs (global meaning) or they integrate their meaning of the situation into their preexisting beliefs or goals. This renewed purpose of rethinking of one's values and setting new goals is critical to this process. If this does not happen, then maladaptive coping occurs, leading to rumination.

Finding meaning in caregiving is underpinned by the existential perspective, a theoretical and philosophical view, which focuses on how people make sense of their existence and assign meaning to it. This perspective on human suffering is necessary before finding that meaning can occur (Frankl 1984; Pearlin et al. 1990; Farran et al. 1997). It is assumed that through suffering the carer can rise above and find and create meaning. This concept of finding meaning has been described as the cognitive transformative process that some caregivers undergo whilst enduring the demands of caregiving, which changes a negative situation into a beneficial and meaningful experience (Farran et al. 1997; Salmon et al. 2005). Viktor Frankl, a prominent figure in psychology and frequently cited in meaning of life research, refers to this as *will to meaning*, arguing that it is a primary and universal human motive (1963). Thus, meaning has to be discovered or found. Frankl's existential perspective suggests that values play an important role in determining how a person deals with difficult situations. In caregiving, finding meaning requires valuing the positive aspect of the caregiving experience and relationship process. Finding meaning offers a different view of the caregiving experience as it includes aspects related to spirituality, personal growth and change, and the search for meaning, and it acknowledges the uniqueness of each caregiver's experience.

Although limited, there has been some research in the area of interventions for finding meaning in caregiving. In a review of the literature, in which meaning and motivation in caregivers of persons with dementia was investigated, finding meaning in caregiving was found to improve caregiver well-being in six studies (Quinn et al. 2010). In an earlier phenomenological study, Butcher and Buckwalter (2002) explore how caregivers find meaning in the caregiving process. Their analysis revealed that the caregivers constructed meaning by recounting memories, living life fully and counting their blessings. Additionally, these researchers suggested that reading narratives written by other caregivers and writing personal experiences and thoughts about caregiving may facilitate the process. In a more recent study, McLennon et al. (2011) suggest that caregivers of spouses with dementia who find meaning through caregiving may experience a partial reduction in the effect of caregiver burden on mental health. It would appear that a caregiver's ability to find meaning in caregiving could potentially affect whether or not they will be able to identify positive aspects of caregiving.

Key Points

- Meaning-focused coping is under-researched.
- Meaning-focused coping can positively impact caregiving experience.

Religious Coping Strategy

Religion is a multifunctional phenomenon, and religious beliefs, attitudes and practices are part of everyday life for many families and caregivers. Religion plays an important role for some families in adapting positively to their caregiving role. There is a growing body of evidence that explores the process of using spiritual and/or religious beliefs as a means of coping in the face of adversity, for example, in trauma and child abuse. Despite the widespread notion that religious and spiritual beliefs help to cope with stress, not much attention has been given to religion as a coping strategy and its influence on health and well-being until relatively recently. Kenneth Pargament, an American psychologist, has written several articles on this subject and is a leading researcher in the field. He argues that religion is another way of coping. According to Pargament (1997), religious coping is defined as a particular sacred means that a person uses to understand and deal with difficult situations. Similarly, Folkman (1997) says religion is an important aspect of meaning-focused coping and argues that under conditions of chronic and severe stress, spirituality and religiosity facilitate positive reappraisals of the difficult situation. Folkman (1997) also states that positive emotions in the coping process are often tied to one's values and beliefs. Thus, religious coping can be a helpful positive adaptive coping strategy. Religious coping can be triggered by situations which push the caregivers beyond their personal and social resources.

Religious coping, however, is far from simple and is regarded as a multifunctional phenomenon that is influenced by different religious groups and cultures (Pargament and Raiya 2007). In Folkman's model, it is not the negative event that determines how well carers adapt but their appraisal of the event and ability to meet the situation's or event's demands. From a sociological perspective, religious belief and practice has and remains a prominent area of research with varying theoretical perspective offered on the subject. The functionalist view of religion offered by anthropologist Malinowski (1954) states that religion performs as a coping mechanism within society in times of emotional stress. Whilst studying Trobriland Islanders over 60 years ago in the Western Pacific, Malinowski identified two types of situations in which religion performs this role – first where the outcome is important but uncontrollable, and thus uncertain, and second in times of crisis. Both these situations resonate with family caregivers even today.

Negative and Positive Religious Coping in Family Carers

Pargament does not assume that all forms of religious coping leads to positive outcomes and he makes a distinction between positive and negative religious coping. Positive religious coping dimension provides comfort, reassurance and an enhanced sense of meaning, whereas negative religious coping dimension reflects a more painful struggle (Pargament et al. 2000). It is argued that the use of adaptive (positive) religious coping can help carers in three main ways – facilitate a restructuring of the carers' beliefs, provide social support via their faith-based communities and provide a greater sense of control over their stressors.

There are several patient-focused studies that demonstrate robust links between positive religious coping and positive physical and mental health outcomes, such as reduced stress and less severe symptoms of depression (Dalmida et al. 2009) and improved quality of life (QoL) in cancers patients (Tarakeshwar et al. 2006), and more specifically faster illness recovery rates/shorter lengths of hospital stay (Contrada et al. 2004). Less frequent are studies on religious coping and its health implications amongst family caregivers. Some studies have focused on religious coping in carers of people with cancer. Mosher et al. (2015) reports that religious coping strategies were commonly used among American caregivers of relatives with advanced lung cancer. Similar results were obtained in a qualitative study of Indian caregivers, who depended on their faith to manage the demands of their relative's cancer and provided a source of strength and contributed to positive life changes (Mehrotra and Sukumar 2007). Similarly, in their study amongst the caregivers of patient with non-metastatic cancer in Western India, Thombre et al. (2010) found that positive religious coping was associated with positive growth. Both studies acknowledged that the results may reflect the dominant Hindu philosophy in India, which emphasises the need to perform positive acts in life to gain good karma and, therefore, end the cycle of reincarnation, i.e., reach moksha. Pearce et al. (2006) indicated that frequent use of negative religious coping strategies amongst caregivers of terminally ill cancer patients was related to more burden, lower QoL and less satisfaction, which also correlated with an increased likelihood of major depressive disorder and anxiety. It is conceivable that religious coping gives purpose and hope to carers, helping them adjust to difficult events by positively reappraising their situation and thus seeing their problems more positively. We will explore personal growth as a result of caregiving in Chapter 5.

Other studies have focused on unanticipated shocking events that abruptly necessitate caregiving for a family member and confronting the family with severe challenges, such as a life-threatening situation (e.g. stroke), that draw the carer to religion as a coping strategy. For example, Gholamzadeh et al. (2014) explored the relationship between religious coping and psychological well-being amongst Iranian caregivers of stroke survivors and reported a significant correlation between positive religious coping and caregivers' psychological well-being. In a study exploring caregiving rewards and coping strategies in caregivers of people with mental illness, the researchers found that a surprising number of carers used increased religiousness and searching for meaning as a coping strategy (Bauer et al. 2013).

Religious Coping and Cultural Difference

Religious beliefs and practice form an important part of culture and individual values and principles. Literature on the use of religious coping in caregivers in the main has concentrated on Western society, although evidence of the adaptive strategy across diverse groups and cultures does exist. Whilst coping strategies may transcend cultures, evidence suggests that there may be some fundamental difference in how these are used. The deployment of religious coping in caregivers may not be uniform. It is well-documented that, in general, women invest in religious participation more than men and that some races tend to be more religious than others, such as African Americans. Several studies have indicated that Black caregivers are more likely to use religious coping resources when dealing with stressful situations compared to Caucasian caregivers (Miltiades and Pruchno 2002; Morano and King 2005; Heo and Koeske 2013). Whilst these studies do not provide a reason for this, a probable explanation is the widely accepted theory that being part of an ethnic minority group, e.g., Afro-Caribbean, leads to higher religious participation than White groups because religion provides a sense of community and cultural identity in a foreign country where feelings of isolation may occur.

Critical to Pargament's theory of religious coping is understanding the function religious resources have in stressful times. A key point here is that a clear distinction needs to be made between claiming that a person has a religious belief and living it with an emotional commitment. This means that it is not just a question of establishing religious beliefs in families and carers, but rather asking how they use their religious beliefs or resources to deal with their caregiving role. For family caregivers attending church and participating in church activities, social support is the primary coping mechanism by which religion helps them to cope. In contrast, for carers who engage in more personal religious coping strategies, religion may reaffirm their values and beliefs and facilitate a positive perspective on the situation.

Since assessing spiritual needs forms a part of the holistic and systematic nursing assessment of patients, their families and carers, addressing these key questions should essentially recognise and respond to the needs of the human spirit. Arguably, this begins with the nurse being sensitive to these needs, picking up clues that may indicate a spiritual need (e.g. religious objects around the home). Care may also include the opportunity for families and carers to express themselves to a sensitive listener or to assess the need for faith support, in which case it may be useful for nurses to refer to a pastoral counsellor, chaplain or other faith groups who will be sensitive to their specific religious backgrounds. Equally important is recognising that for some carers religious struggles or doubts (negative religious coping) may be harmful, leading to poor mental health; for example, in doubting Gods' existence as a Muslim, which is not acceptable in Islamic culture, the carer may experience alienation and loneliness, which may lead to depression (Pargement and Raiya 2007). Equally, the inability of the family carer to attend religious services due to their caregiving demands may lead to isolation and disapproval from the religious community, which may lead to further distress. This emphasises the need for nurses, when caring for families, to be aware of these potential struggles in times of crisis when their faith may be questioned and to be aware of the challenges that different religions may require of an individual. Research highlights the need for nurses to be culturally sensitive and to understand the importance of religion as a coping resource in certain groups of caregivers.

Religious coping is an important consideration in the caregiving process and one that nurses need to be acutely aware of, and it may be a useful resource for some families to draw on in time of acute crisis. Either way the social or the spiritual aspects of religion seem to have a buffering effect on family caregivers' stress levels. It can also play an important part in the interpretation and management of traumatic events and in the promotion of resiliency. Having a greater understanding of religious coping and its role in the caregiving process can help provide better ways to assisting racially diverse caregivers in dealing with the struggles of caregiving. It would appear that positive religious coping more than negative religious coping significantly affects family carers' psychological well-being. Further research is needed to establish the important issues that influence religious coping and the positive and negative impact on caregiving. There is also a need to understand how family caregivers draw on their faith to help manage these demands, and the role of religious coping in enhancing carers' psychological well-being needs to be considered in family intervention programmes.

Key Points

- Religious coping is a multifunctional phenomenon influenced by religion and culture.
- Religious coping is an important unrecognised coping resource.
- Religious coping can be positive (adaptive) or negative (maladaptive).

Humour

Humour, fundamentally a social phenomenon, is an emotion familiar to all of us that is elicited by a particular set of cognitive appraisals that a situation is funny or amusing. Freud (1960) touted that humour may be the most effective of all coping or defence mechanisms; however, there is little empirical evidence to support this notion. Humour as a coping strategy, defined as the propensity to utilise humour as a method for coping with stressful or demanding situation, is often used to cope with the caregiving task. The literature on the use of humour as a coping strategy in caregivers is limited. Some researchers have looked at the effectiveness of humour in mitigating caregiver stress (Abel 1998; Parrish and Quinn 1999; Reiger 2004). Others have found that humour, laughing and joking, was used as a way of coping by carers of stroke survivors (O'Connell and Baker 2004) and Alzheimer's disease (Tan and Schneider 2009) and that it significantly impacted caregivers' well-being (Buffum and Brod 1998). Parrish and Quinn (1999) maintain that humour and laughter are the unsung heroes of coping for caregivers. They also maintain that humour helps carers survive difficult and painful situations along with providing a well-deserved, albeit temporary, peace of mind. Bethea et al. (2000) also argue that humour is more than 'funny stories' about caregiving and that it serves as several communicative functions for long-term caregivers; as a comfortable way to share personal and often sensitive information, humour acts as a means to explain how or why they thought, felt or acted in a certain way and that finally it can serve to communicate an unresolved caregiving conflict or concern. Humour may even provide a sense of escapism or create a sense of distancing from the realities of caregiving, which may enable the carer to explore alternative solutions to their problems, and laughter can improve a carers' mood and overall sense of happiness. According to Lefcourt and Martin (1986), humour may alter a person's perception of the situation, making the situation less stressful and arousing. In terms of transactional theory of emotion and coping (Lazarus and Folkman 1984), the effectiveness of humour can be explained by caregivers positively appraising their stressful situation. In addition, from a physiological perspective, the effects of humour on the neuroendocrine system are well known, helping to explain the buffering effect on stress, i.e., most notably the effect on the release of endorphins (acts on the body in a similar way to opiates) which relaxes the body. From a spiritual perspective, Viktor Frankl (1984), in a narrative of his imprisonment in a Nazi concentration camp, identifies humour as 'one of the soul's weapons in the fight for self-preservation' (p. 63).

Although the use of appropriate humour is an important element of human well-being and it may be at the core of survival for some carers, it is crucial to recognise that humour requires boundaries, especially when focused on sensitive issues, and thus requires careful assessment as to when and with whom it is used. Equally, cultural differences and perception need to be considered. Whilst humour may not solve a problem, it can ease or relieve tension, but when used negatively, it can act as a screen and thus block communication. Humour has been found to be an important influence in the levels of hope (Herth 1990;

Miller 1991). Humour is one coping strategy that is often used by individuals who are high in hope (Parrish and Quinn 1999; Snyder 1994; Vilaythong et al. 2003).

Hope as a Coping Strategy

Hope is a common, universal human experience that is difficult to deconstruct. It is highly individual and has the capacity to act in a mysterious way. It is a crucial factor in helping carers cope with uncertainty and difficult circumstances that caregiving conjures up. It also enables carers to envisage a future. Hope is important in the adjustment process following illness, trauma and disability and is both an affective and powerful cognitive coping strategy for caregivers. Additionally, interventions can be targeted at hope; we will return to this later in Chapter 6. Caregiving brings with it the need for hope, and for this key reason the following section will explore the concept of hope with the aim of helping nurses to understand the nature of hope and the role of hope in the coping process.

Definition of Hope

The literature does not offer a consensus on hope, with varying theological and philosophical definitions ranging from simple wishful thinking to theoretical constructs, but all seem to include the idea of a positive, future orientation. Several researchers have made attempts to define hope over the past 30 years or so, and what seems evident is that its complex subjective nature makes it impossible to draw a simple definition. Miller (1986, p. 52) provides an operational definition of hope:

> An anticipation of a future which is good and based upon: mutuality (relationships with others), a sense of personal competence, coping ability, psychological well-being, purpose and meaning in life, as well as a sense of 'the possible'.

Whilst others have identified hope as a 'process of anticipation that involves the interaction of thinking, acting, feeling and relating, and is directed towards a future fulfilment that is personally meaningful' (Stephenson 1991, p. 1459). More recently, family therapist Pauline Boss (2006) conceives hope as a positive belief in a future good, that suffering can stop, and the belief in the expectation of future comfort. There is a general understanding that hope is in all of us and hope is not just about optimism for the future but is also about making and enacting realistic plans to attain future objectives. But without hope there is despair. Hope seems to be closely linked to meaning and to spirituality and faith, although it is argued that hope is not the same as faith. For example, Boss (2006, p. 177) states that 'without meaning, there is no hope and without hope, there is no meaning'. In a similar vein, Viktor Frankl discovered, whilst being held captive in Nazi concentration camps in the Second World War, that *where there is no hope, life ceases* (Frankl 1984).

Despite the varying definitions, hope, in essence, is the overall perception that one's goals can be met. Four main components of hope have been proposed (Farran et al. 1995; Snyder 2000):

1. Hope is focused on the future.
2. Hope anticipates that the future will be better than the present.
3. Hope has both cognitive and affective aspects.
4. A hopeful person believes that the object of their hopes can be realised.

Theoretical Perspectives

Over the past two decades, several theoretical models of hope have been developed which have influenced researchers in several fields of practice, including nursing. Whilst it is beyond the scope of this book to explore these in detail, we provide some exposure of the commonly cited models which have clinical application and how they offer explanations for the role of hope in coping. The psychologist Charles R. Snyder's (Snyder 1994) cognitive goal-directed hope theory has been widely researched and tested and often described as a trilogy of hope that consists of three components – goals, pathways and sense of agency. For Snyder, hope is a positive motivated state that comprises these three distinct but interrelated elements (Snyder and Lopez 2007). Snyder conceptualises hope as a goal-directed cognitive process which reflects people's motivation and capacity to strive towards personally relevant goals (Snyder 1994). According to the theory, goals must be perceived as being attainable with pathways (way power) or workable routes towards goal achievement evident by statements such as *I can find a way to get this done* and sense of agency (willpower) or the person's perceived capacity to initiate and sustain goal-directed efforts evident by statements such as *I can do this*. Thus, Snyder's hope has two aspects: the individual's belief that a favourable outcome is possible and the individual's ability to visualise how that outcome will come about. Both these components have been validly measured, e.g., using the hope scale (Snyder et al. 1996). Snyder (2000) also argues that hope has three necessary ingredients:

1. Goal-oriented thoughts – non-random human behaviours are directed by some goal, either short term or long term.
2. Goals need to be of sufficient value to the individual so as to occupy conscious thought.
3. Goals should be attainable yet challenging in nature – goals that are 100% likely to be achieved do not give people hope.

Based on the key principle of the interactive development of pathways and agency, in order to achieve goals, people need to generate plausible routes. This may involve one or several pathways. When an obstacle arises, alternative pathways should be created. According to Snyder (1996), *high-hope individuals* typically can clearly conceptualise their goals, envision one major pathway to a desired goal, can generate alternative pathways, especially when the original one is blocked, and perceive that they will actively employ pathways in pursuit of their goals. Research indicates that people with high levels of hope believe that they are capable of finding alternative ways and can be very effective at creating alternative routes (Snyder et al. 2000). Thus, hopeful caregivers may become more goal oriented in an effort to seek alternative pathways to overcome their challenges.

Snyder's theory has attracted some critics over the years, some arguing that it neglects the social context and personal influences in the agency or willpower. Lazarus (1999) also challenges the agency component by arguing that we can hope even when we are helpless in affecting the outcome. Despite this, Folkman and Greer (2000) identified Snyder's concept of hope as a variable that influences an individual's secondary appraisal, i.e., the extent to which a situation can be controlled or changed by an individual's appraisal of the stressor. Snyder's explanatory model has led to the development of specific interventions designed to systematically increase hope in individuals.

The American nurse researcher Kaye Herth has also been influential in shaping hope theory. Her model of hope, like Snyder, emphasises the cognitive aspect of hope and views hope as a motivational and cognitive attribute that is necessary to initiate and sustain action towards goal attainment. Based on studies with cancer patients and older people living in nursing homes, Herth (2000) identified three dimensions of hope that correlate with patients' psychosocial functioning: (a) cognitive–temporal (beliefs that a person can obtain goals), (b) affective–behavioural (reflecting a person's confidence in their plans to achieve the goals), and (c) affiliative–contextual (an individual's perceived social support, spiritual support, and sense of belongingness). The first two components resonate with Snyder's agency and pathway component respectively.

Dufault and Martocchio (1985), based on interviews with older people with cancer, produced a multidimensional concept of hope, which includes philosophical, theological, sociological, psychological and nursing perspectives of hope. The researchers defined hope as 'multidimensional dynamic life force characterized by a confident yet uncertain expectation of achieving future good, which to the hoping person is realistically possible and personally significant' (Dufault and Martocchio 1985, p. 380). Within their conceptual model, two spheres of hope are identified: particularised hope and generalised hope. Particularised hope is focused on specific hope goals or a wish, whilst generalised hope has a broad outlook that makes life worthwhile. Both these spheres operate together. Dufault and Martocchio (1985) also describe six domains which depict the experience of hope: affective, cognitive, behavioural, affiliative, temporal and contextual.

Hope, in the context of nursing, is argued by many theorists to be one of the fundamental ingredients of caring. In Jean Watson's Caring theory (2012), which provides nurses with guidance for providing care to ease not just the patient suffering but their families, hope is an essential component. Within Jean Watson's caring theory, 10 primary carative factors (renamed later as 'caritas processes') form the basis for caring, and 3 form the 'philosophical foundation' for the science of caring. The installation of hope is one of these three. Thus, hope is considered a significant component in the caritas process (caring process), recognising the essential value of hope for both carative and the curative processes and the positive effects on healing and alleviating suffering.

The philosopher Milton Mayeroff (1925–1979), who has informed many nursing theorist including Watson, in his classic work On Caring (1971) wrote that hope is the seventh (of eight) essential caring ingredient, and stated that hope is "An expression of the plentitude of the present, alive with a sense of a possible" (p. 26). Interestingly Mayeroff does not differentiate between families or patients when he refers to caring, but states 'appropriate others' referring to all that require care.

Caregiver Literature on Hope

There is increasing recognition in the literature that hope is a unique and important influence on the adaptation to illness and promoting wellness. The published studies of hope and family caregivers have been both descriptive and exploratory and carried out in a variety of family settings ranging from caregivers of persons with dementia, cancer and chronic illness to those caring for people receiving critical care. Most support the notion that hope is an important factor in caregiving. In Duggleby et al.'s (2010) meta-synthesis of hope experiences of family caregivers of members with chronic illness, hope was found to be an important factor in all the studies regardless of age, relationship, or setting. A key shared finding in this meta-synthesis was the transitional refocusing by family caregivers from a difficult present to a positive future. In addition, for family caregivers whose coping strategies were more day to day, shorter time frames for defining future were envisaged, whereas for caregivers who were contemplating a future for more than a day, this was difficult. In a later study, Utne et al. (2013) suggest that family carers and patients' level of hope are important determinants of caregiver burden and that family caregivers with lower levels of hope represent a high-risk group for higher levels of caregiver burden. Findings from this study suggest that family carers' and patients' level of hope are important determinants of caregiver burden.

Some studies have investigated the relation between hope and adaptive coping and have found a negative correlation with anxiety and depression. In a study exploring the role of hope in adapting to uncertainty in 546 caregivers of children with Down syndrome, the researchers concluded that having hope in the face of uncertainty is important in adaptation to stressors (Truitt et al. 2012). Similarly, hope has been found to support parents as they care for their children with a life-limiting or life-threatening illness (Kylma and Juvakka 2007; Bally et al. 2014). Hunsaker et al. (2014) in their study not only established the reliability and validity of the HHS in families of cognitively impaired individuals but they also concluded that the families in their study can maintain hope in the face of a potentially progressive illness regardless of cognitive status. These studies provide further evidence of the importance of fostering hope in supporting families and caregivers.

Key Points

- Hope is a basic human response regardless of age, gender or ethnicity but highly individual.
- Hope theory relates to the perceived expectation that goals can be achieved.
- Hope is a vital personal adaptive coping resource.
- Further research into hope experiences in family caregivers is needed.

Coping Ability: Sense of Coherence and General Resistance Resources

So far, we have explored a variety of coping strategies that a family caregiver may use in their carer's role. The ability to use a variety of coping strategies and the most effective strategy in different stressful situations is explained by the American-Israeli medical sociologist Aaron Antonovsky as SOC, a core component of his salutogenic theory. Over 30 years ago, Antonovsky introduced his salutogenesis theory as an alternative view of health from the pathogenic orientation (i.e. focusing on origins of disease) underpinning the biomedical world, which tends to a cause and effect relationship of disease and illness. Salutogenesis means the origins (genesis) of health (saluto). This reflected at that time a paradigm shift from thinking about what made people sick to why people stayed healthy. Antonovsky's idea for his theory came from studying women who had survived concentration camps during the Second World War and despite that stayed healthy. As to why this occurred led to the development of the salutogenic theory of health (Antonovsky 1979). Antonovsky focused on the underlying social constructs, in other words, the bigger picture, to explain the factors which maintain or promote human health rather than just factors that cause disease-related health problems. The salutogenic orientation views individuals on a *health–disease continuum* and considers that all have the ability to move along the health continuum in either direction, and tension and strain are viewed as potentially health-promoting. This philosophical orientation is a departure from the view that stress events can result in disease as articulated by early stress theorists, such as Hans Selye. Antonovsky argues that stressors are omnipresent or continually present and that they create tension. In salutogenesis, stress occurs when demands outweigh a carer's resources, resulting in a movement towards a lower level of health. Salutogenesis is a stress resource–orientated concept, which focuses on resources and maintains and improves the movement towards health (Lindstrom and Eriksson 2005). For Antonovsky, humans are open, self-regulating systems, and people with high levels of health are high self-regulators. As the model focuses on successful coping, it would seem an appropriate model to focus on to help explain how some caregivers cope and remain healthy whilst other do not and to present as a new way of thinking about the management of stressors.

Antonovsky created two key concepts in his theory of salutogenesis – general resistance resources (GRRs) and *sense of coherence*. GRRs are described as any characteristic that can facilitate effective tension management, where tension is caused by the stressors (Antonovsky 1987). Antonovsky classified these resources into different groups, but for the purpose of this book, these can be viewed as personal resources (e.g. self-esteem and cognitive ability to cope) and general psychosocial resources (e.g. social support and culture). According to Antonovsky, if stressors can be coped with successfully, the individual moves in a positive direction of the health–disease continuum, and, if not, a state of stress occurs and the individual moves to the negative side of the continuum. Antonovsky calls the individual's position on this continuum *sense of coherence* (Antonovsky 1979); see Figure 4.1. Antonovsky (1979) explained SOC as a generalised, long-lasting way of seeing the world and one's life in it. Three intertwined life experiences or components shape the concept of SOC – *comprehensibility*, the ability of people to understand what happens around them or understand the challenges; *manageability*, the extent to which they are able to manage the situation on their own or through significant others in their social network, i.e., resources; and *meaningfulness*, the ability to find meaning in the situation and the ability to identify

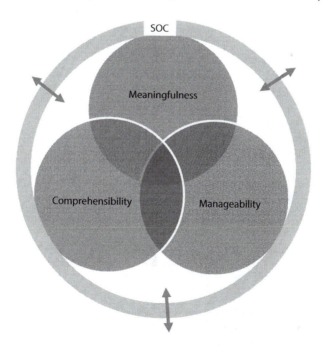

Figure 4.1 Sense of coherence (SOC) and its interrelated components.

challenges that are worth devoting energy to in order to deal with them successfully. Antonovsky emphasised the third component, meaningfulness, influenced by the work of Viktor Frankl on meaning, as the most important component.

A SOC relates to the way a person views the world and how he or she assesses and copes with stressful situations using these available resources (Antonovsky 1979). Thus, a carer's appraisal of the level of resources and capacity to employ these resources have consequences on how they cope and on their level of health. In other words, a carer's health is dependent on their ability to cope, the number and strength of the resources (GRRs) they use to help them cope and their SOC. If a carer lacks GRRs, in effect, this reduces their SOC and vice versa, as indicated by the outer circle and arrows in Figure 4.1. Crucially for Antonovsky, the existence of resources is not sufficient to deal with the challenges that life throws at us, such as caregiving; rather, the ability to use them is more important. For Reker and Wong (1988), an SOC involves having an integrated and consistent understanding of self, others and life. This sense of coherence and purpose provide insights into how a carer perceives their existence. However, Antonovsky's salutogenic theory is not the only means of explaining positive health, as there are other concepts we have discussed, such as resilience, that help us to understand coping.

McCubbin et al. (1996) regarded SOC as a cognitive process in which individuals and families called upon their available resources to manage the accumulation of family stressors and strains. Time, an important influence on SOC, is developmental (i.e. developing throughout the life course). So over time, experiences that facilitate the development of these three components foster a strong SOC (i.e. during childhood and young adulthood), and the stronger the SOC, the more a person's ability to employ cognitive, affective and instrumental strategies that lead to coping and well-being (Antonovsky 1987). Thus, as family caregivers advance in age, understanding their range of abilities, confidence and awareness increases (Mizuno et al. 2012). It is conceivable that increasing age may be a protective or mediating factor in caregiver stress. Salutogenic theory recognises a caregiver's resources for coping with caregiving, and a caregiver with a strong or high SOC would have a greater coping capacity with more available resources for choosing adaptive successful coping strategies. A caregiver with a higher SOC is expected to have a greater ability to manage stress, whereas a low SOC would mean that family caregivers would find their situation less comprehensible, more difficult to manage and less meaningful with fewer resources to adapt to their situation. Over the course of time, caregivers may come to make sense of the world, and although philosophically different from life events, as discussed in Chapter 3, the notion of time and experience are undoubtedly important for understanding caregiving.

In order for nurses to be able to promote health in family caregivers and understand how they use their resources to maintain health, a greater understanding of caregiver resources to health is required. Antonovsky's salutogenic theory offers insight into why some caregivers cope better than others. Although the salutogenic model does not refer to a specific coping strategy, it refers to the factors that can be used to cope with stressors. Given that carers' SOC can be manipulated and be pushed towards health, it would seem pertinent for nurses to be aware of the importance of SOC. The salutogenic model can offer and direct attention to interventions which enhance their SOC. This may include adding or extending coping resources (factors), identifying what factors or strategies are currently functioning well and, finally, promoting these factors. Arguably, nurses who strengthen carers' SOC promote wellness and foster carers' ability to stay well or get well, which are important aspects of nursing care.

Antonovsky (1987), following the publication of his salutogenic theory, developed a scale to measure the concept of SOC, called the coherence scale SOC-29 (29 items), and the short version SOC-13 (13 items), which comprises three subscales: meaningfulness, comprehensibility and manageability. This scale has been widely used across many settings and has been found to be a reliable, valid and cross-culturally applicable instrument that is able to measure how individuals manage stressful situations and stay well (Lindstrom and Eriksson 2005). Several quantitative studies have explored SOC using this scale amongst a variety of caregiver populations including caregivers of persons with stroke (Forsberg-Warleby et al. 2002; Chumbler et al. 2008; Van Puymbroec et al. 2008), schizophrenia (Suresky et al. 2008; Mizuno et al. 2012) and dementia (Andrén and Elmsåhl 2008; Pretorius et al. 2009; Stenletten et al. 2014). These research findings all seem to suggest that a strong SOC buffers against the negative effects of caregiving (burden and depression) and is associated with better coping abilities. Because SOC is linked to and influences a person's QoL, some caregiver studies have explored this correlation and found that family caregivers with high SOC scores enjoy a high QoL (Mizuno et al. 2012).

Key Points

- Salutogenic concepts of personal and environmental resources and SOC help caregivers to cope.
- SOC can be seen as developmental and determined by life experiences.
- A carer with a strong SOC is more likely to cope.

Chapter Summary

Clearly, coping is a complex dynamic process and is an important topic in helping to understand how families and caregivers cope with their caregiving role. Coping strategies play an important role in the caregiving process. Coping is influenced by the intrinsic qualities of the carer and the availability of external resources. Whilst there is no categorical evidence as to which coping strategy is most effective, a carer will prefer to use a strategy that reduces stress. This chapter has mainly focused on the fundamentals of the coping process, which would apply to any family caregiver. We have examined various coping strategies that may be used by family caregivers. No single style of coping is adaptive to all situations or events. It would appear that if family caregivers use an appropriate coping strategy based upon their appraisal of the demands of the situation, they are more likely to experience success in their efforts to manage the situation. Families and caregivers differ in their access to and use of coping strategies in coping with their caregiving demands. Understanding the various ways that family caregivers cope with stress is critical if nurses and other healthcare professionals are to support them in their caregiving role. Further research is warranted to explore and interpret contextual factors such as age, gender, ethnicity and degrees of caregiving responsibilities that may influence the caregiver's choice of coping strategy.

References

Abel MH. (1998) Interaction of humour and gender in modulating relationships between stress and outcome. *Journal of Psychology* 132(3): 267–276.

Almberg B, Grafström B and Winblad B. (1997) Major strain and coping strategies as reported by family members who care for aged demented relatives *Journal of Advanced Nursing* 26: 683–691.

Andrén S and Elmståhl S. (2008) The relationship between caregiver burden, caregivers' perceived health and their sense of coherence in caring for elders with dementia. *Journal of Clinical Nursing* 17(6): 790–799.

Antonovsky A. (1979) *Health, Stress and Coping.* San Francisco, CA: Jossey-Bass.

Antonovsky A. (1987) *Unravelling the Mystery of Health: How People Manage Stress and Stay Well.* San Francisco, CA: Jossey-Boss.

Bally JMGT, Duggleby W, Holtslander L, Mpofu C, Spurr S, Thomas R and Wright K. (2014) Keeping hope possible: A grounded theory study of the hope experience of parental caregivers who children have terminal cancers. *Cancer Nursing* 37(5): 363–372.

Bauer R, Sterzinger L, Koepke F and Spiessl H. (2013) Rewards of caregiving and coping strategies of caregivers of patients with mental illness. *Psychiatric Services* 64(2): 185–188.

Bautista RED and Erwin PA. (2013) Analyzing depression coping strategies of patients with epilepsy: A preliminary study. *Seizure* 22(9): 686–691.

Bethea LS, Travis SS and Pecchioni L. (2000) Family cargivers's use of humor in conveying information about caring for dependent older adults. *Health Communication* 12(4): 361–376.

Bond AE, Draeger CRL, Mandleco B and Donnelly M. (2003) Needs of family members of patients with severe traumatic brain injury: Implications for evidence-based practice. *Critical Care Nurse* 23(4): 63–72.

Boss P. (2006) *Loss Trauma and Resilience.* New York: W.W. Norton & Company.

Buffum MD and Brod M. (1998) Humor and well-being in spouse caregivers of patients with Alzheimer's disease. *Applied Nursing Research* 11(1): 12–18.

Butcher HK and Buckwalter KC. (2002) Exasperations as blessings: Meaning-making in family caregiving. *Journal of Aging and Identity* 7: 113–132.

Carver CS, Scheier MF and Weinhtraub JK. (1989) Assessing coping strategies: A theoretically based approach. *Journal of Personality and Social Psychology* 56(2): 267–283.

Case DO, Andrews JE, Johnson JD and Allard SL. (2005) Avoiding verse seeking: The relationship of information seeking to avoidance, blunting, coping, dissonance, and related concepts. *Journal of Medical Library Association* 93(3): 353–362.

Chumbler NR, Rittman MR and Wu SS. (2008) Associations in sense of coherence and depression in caregivers of stroke survivors across 2 years. *Journal of Behavioral Health Services and Research* 35(2): 226–234.

Contrada RJ, Goyal TM, Cather C, Rafalson L, Idler EL and Krause TJ. (2004) Psychosocial factors in outcome of heart surgery: The impact of religious involvement and depressive symptoms. *Health Psychology* 23: 227–238.

Cooper C, Katona C, Orrell M and Livingston G. (2008) Coping strategies, anxiety and depression in caregivers of people with Alzheimer's disease. *International Journal of Geriatric Psychiatry* 23: 929–936.

Cotton SM, McCann TV, Gleeson JF, Crisp K, Murphy BP and Lubman DI. (2013) Coping strategies in carers of young people with a first episode of psychosis. *Schizophrenia Research* 146(1–3): 118–124.

Dalmida SG, Holstad MM, Dilorio C and Laderman G. (2009) Spiritual well-being, depressive symptoms and immune status amongst women with HIV/AIDS. *Women Health* 49: 119–143.

Dufault K and Martocchio BC. (1985) Hope: Its spheres and dimensions. *Nursing Clinics of North America* 20(2): 379–391.

Duggleby WD, Holstlander L, Kylma J, Duncan V, Hammond C and Williams A. (2010) Metasynthesis of the hope experience of family caregivers of persons with chronic illness. *Qualitative Health Research* 20(2): 148–158.

D'Zurilla TJ. (1986) *Problem-Solving Therapy: A Social Competence Approach to Clinical Intervention.* New York: Springer Publishing Company.

Endler NS and Parker JDA. (1990) The multidimensional assessment of coping: A critical evaluation. *Journal of Personality and Social Psychology* 58: 844–854.

Farran CJ, Herth KA and Popivich JM. (1995) *Hope and Hopelessness: Critical Clinical Constructs.* Thousand Oaks, CA: Sage.

Farran CJ, Miller BH, Kaufman JE and Davis L. (1997) Race, finding meaning, and caregiver distress. *Journal of Aging and Health* 9: 316–333.

Folkman S and Lazarus RS. (1980). An analysis of coping in a middle-aged community sample. *Journal of Health and Social Behaviour* 21: 219–239.

Folkman S. (1997) Positive psychological states and coping with severe stress. *Social Science & Medicine* 45(8): 1207–1221.

Folkman S. (2008) The case of positive emotions in the stress process. *Anxiety, Stress and Coping* 2(1): 3–14.

Folkman S and Greer S. (2000) Promoting psychological well-being in the face of serious illness: When theory, research and practice inform each other. *Psycho-Oncology* 9: 11–19.

Folkman S, Lazarus RS, Gruen RJ and DeLongis A. (1986) Appraisal, coping, health status and psychological symptoms. *Journal of Personality and Social Psychology* 50: 571–579.

Forsberg-Wärleby G, Möller A and Blomstrand C. (2002) Spouses of first-ever stroke victims: Sense of coherence in the first phase after stroke. *Journal of Rehabilitation Medicine* 34(3): 128–133.

Frankl VE. (1984) *Man's Search for Meaning.* New York: Pocket Books.

Freud S. (1960) *Jokes and Their Relation to the Unconscious* (trans. J. Strachey, Ed.). New York: Norton.

Fulbrook P, Allan D, Carrol S and Dawson D. (1999) On the receiving end: Experiences of being a relative in critical care, part 1. *Nursing in Critical Care* 4: 138–145.

Gaeeni M, Farahani MA, Seyedfatemi N and Mohammadi N. (2015) Informational support to family members of intensive care unit patients: The perspectives of families and nurses. *Global Journal of Health Science* 7(2): 8–19.

Gholamzadeh S, Hamid TA, Basri H, Sharif F and Ibrahim R. (2014) Religious coping and psychological well-being among Iranian stroke caregivers. *Iran Journal of Nursing Midwifery Research* 19(5): 478–484.

Heo GJ and Koeske G. (2013) The role of religious coping and race in Alzheimer's disease caregiving. *Journal of Applied Gerontology* 32(5): 582–604.

Herth K. (1990) The relationship between hope, coping styles concurrent losses, and setting to grief resolution in the elderly widow(er). *Research in Nursing Health* 13(2): 109–117.

Herth KA. (2000) Enhancing hope in people with a first recurrence of cancer. *Journal of Advanced Nursing* 32: 1431–1441.

Herth KA. (2001) Development and implementation of a hope intervention program. *Oncology Nursing Forum* 28(10): 1009–1017.

Holahan CJ, Moos RH and Schaefer JA. (1996) Coping, stress, resistance, and growth: Conceptualising adaptive functioning. In: M. Zeidner and N. S. Endler (Eds.) *Handbook of Coping: Theory, Research, Applications*. New York: John Wiley & Sons, Inc., pp. 24–43.

Huang MF, Huang WH, Su YC, Hou SY, Chen HM, Yeh YC and Chen CS. (2015) Coping strategy and caregiver burden among caregivers of patients with dementia. *American Journal of Alzheimer's Disorders and Other Dementias* 30(7): 694–698.

Hunsaker AE, Terhorst L, Gentry A and Lingler JH. (2014) Measuring hope among families impacted by cognitive impairment. *Dementia*. doi:10.1177/1471301214531590.

Kim Y, Schulz R and Carver CS. (2007) Benefit finding in the cancer caregiving experience. *Psychosomatic Medicine* 69: 283–291.

Kylma J and Juvakka T. (2007) Hope in parents of adolescents with cancer: Factors endangering and engendering parental hope. *European Journal of Oncology Nursing* 11(3): 262–271.

Lazarus RS. (1966) *Psychological Stress and the Coping Process*. New York: McGraw-Hill.

Lazarus RS. (1999) Hope: An emotion and a vital coping resource against despair. *Social Research* 6(2): 653–678.

Lazarus RS and Folkman S. (1984) *Stress Appraisal and Coping*. New York: Springer.

Lefcourt HM and Martin RA. (1986) *Humor and Life Stress: Antidote to Adversity*. New York: Springer-Verlag.

Lindstrom B and Eriksson M. (2005) Salutogenesis. *Journal of Epidemiology and Community Health* 59: 440–442.

Malinowski B. (1954) *Magic, Science and Religion and Other Essays*. New York: Anchor Books.

Maslow AH. (1963) The need to know and the fear of knowing. *Journal of General Psychology* 68(1): 111–125.

Mattsson A. (1972) Long-term physical illness in childhood: A challenge to psychosocial adaptation. *Pediatrics* 50(5): 801–811.

Mayeroff M. (1971) *On Caring*. New York: Harper and Row.

McCubbin HI, Thompson EA, Thompson AI and Fromer JE. (1996) The sense of coherence: A historical and future perspective. *Israeli Journal of Medical Science* 32(3–4): 170–178.

McLennona SM, Habermanna B and Riceb M. (2011) Finding meaning as a mediator of burden on the health of caregivers of spouses with dementia. *Aging & Mental Health* 15(4): 522–530.

Mehrotra S and Sukumar P. (2007) Sources of strength perceived by females caring for relatives diagnosed with cancer: An exploratory study from India. *Supportive Care in Cancer* 15(12): 1357–1366.

Miller J. (1986) Inspiring hope. *American Journal of Nursing* 85: 22–25.

Miller JF. (1991) Developing and maintaining hope in families of the critically ill. *AACN Clinical Issues in Critical Care Nursing* 2: 307–365.

Miltiades H and Pruchno R. (2002) The effect of religious coping on caregiving appraisals of mothers of adults with developmental disabilities. *The Gerontologist* 42(1): 82–91.

Mizuno E, Iwasaki M, Sakai I and Kamizawa N. (2012) Sense of coherence and quality of life in family caregivers of persons with schizophrenia living in the community. *Archives of Psychiatric Nursing* 26(2): 296–306.

Moos RH and Billings AG. (1982) Conceptualizing and measuring coping resources and processes. In: L. Goldberger and S. Brezitz (Eds.) *Handbook of Stress Theoretical and Clinical Aspects.* New York: Free Press, pp. 212–230.

Morano CL and King D. (2005) Religiosity as a mediator of caregiver well-being: Does ethnicity make a difference? *Journal of Gerontological Social Work* 45(1/2): 69–84.

Mosher CE., Ott ME., Hanna N., Jallal SI and Champion VL. (2015) Coping with physical and psychological symptoms: a qualitative study of advanced lung cancers patient's and their family caregivers. Support Cancer Care 23: 2053–2060.

Nolan MR, Grant G and Keady J. (1996) *Understanding Family Care: A Multidimensional Model of Caring and Coping.* Buckingham, United Kingdom: Open University Press.

O'Connell B and Baker L. (2004) Managing as carers of stroke survivors. *International Journal of Nursing Practice* 10(3): 121–126.

Onwumere J, Bebbington P and Kuipers E. (2011) Family interventions in early psychosis: Specificity and effectiveness. *Epidemiology and Psychiatric Science* 20(2): 113–119.

Pargament KI. (1997) *The Psychology of Religion and Coping: Theory, Research and Practice.* New York: Guilford Publications.

Pargament KI, Koenig HG and Perez L. (2000) The many methods of religious coping: Development and initial validation of the RCOPE. *Journal of Clinical Psychology* 56(4): 519–543.

Pargament KI and Raiya HA. (2007) A decade of research on the psychology of religion and coping. *Psyke and Logos* 28: 742–766.

Park CL and Folkman S. (1997) Meaning in the context of stress and coping. *Review of General Psychology* 1(2): 115–144.

Parrish MM and Quinn P. (1999) Laughing your way to peace of mind: How a little humor helps caregivers survive. *Clinical Social Work Journal* 27(2): 203–211.

Pearce MJ, Singer JL and Prigerson HG. (2006) Religious coping among caregivers of terminally ill cancer patients. *Journal of Health Psychology* 11(5): 743–759.

Pearlin LI, Mullan JT, Semple SJ and Skaff MM. (1990) Caregiving, and the stress process: An overview of concepts and their measures. *The Gerontologist* 30: 583–594.

Pearlin LI and Scholer C. (1978) The structure of coping. *Journal of Health Social Behaviour* 19: 1–21.

Pretorius C, Walker S and Heyns PM. (2009) Sense of coherence amongst male caregivers in dementia: A South African perspective. *Dementia* 8(1): 79–94.

Quinn C, Clare L and Woods RT. (2010) The impact of motivation and meanings on the wellbeing of caregivers of people with dementia: A systematic review. *International Psychogeriatrics* 22: 43–55.

Reker GT, Peacock EJ and Wang PTP. (1987) Meaning and purpose of life and well-being a life span perspective. *Journal of Gerontology* 42: 44–49.

Reker GT and Wong PTP. (1988) Aging as an individual process: Toward a theory of personal meaning. In: J. E. Birren and V. L. Bengston (Eds.) *Emergent Theories of Aging.* New York: Springer, pp. 214–246.

Rieger A. (2004) Explorations of the functions of humor and other types of fun among families of children with disabilities. *Research and Practice for Persons with Severe Disabilities* 29(3): 194–209.

Salmon JR, Kwak J, Acquaviva KD, Brandt K and Egan KA. 2005. Transformative aspects of caregiving at life's end. *Journal of Pain and Symptom Management* 29: 121–129.

Snyder CJ and Lopez SJ. (2007) *Positive Psychology: The Scientific and Practical Explorations of Human Strengths.* London, UK: Sage.

Snyder CM, Fauth E, Wanzek J, Piercy KW, Norton MC, Corcoran C, Rabins PV et al. (2015) Dementia caregivers' coping strategies and their relationship to health and well-being: The Cache County Study. *Aging & Mental Health* 19(5): 390–399.

Snyder CR. (1994) *The Psychology of Hope: You can Get There from Here.* New York: Free Press.

Snyder CR. (1996) To hope, to lose, and to hope again. *Journal of Personal and Interpersonal Loss* 1: 1–16.

Snyder CR. (2000) The past and possible futures of hope. *Journal of Social and Clinical Psychology* 19: 11–28.

Snyder CR, Sympson SC, Ybasco FC, Borders TF, Babyak MA and Higgins RL. (1996) Development and validation of the state hope scale. *Journal of Personality and Social Psychology* 70: 321–335.

Snyder CR, Ilardi S, Michael ST and Cheavens J. (2000) Hope theory: Updating a common process for psychological change. In: C.R. Snyder and R.E. Ingram (Eds.), *Handbook of Psychological Change: Psychotherapy Processes and practices for the 21st Century.* New York: John Wiley & Sons.

Stensletten K, Bruvik F, Espehaug B and Drageset J. (2014) Burden of care, social support, and sense of coherence in elderly caregivers living with individuals with symptoms of dementia. *Dementia*, first published on December 18, 2014.

Stephenson C. (1991) The concept of hope revisited for nursing. *Journal of Advanced Nursing* 16: 1456–1461.

Suresky MJ, Zauszniewski JA and Bekhet AK. (2008) Sense of coherence and quality of life in women family members of the seriously mentally ill. *Issues in Mental Health Nursing* 29: 265–278.

Tan T and Schneider MA. (2009) Humor as a coping strategy for adult-child caregivers of individuals with Alzheimer's disease. *Geriatric Nursing* 30(6): 397–408.

Tarakeshwar N, Vanderweker LC, Paulk E, Pearce MJ, Kasl SV and Pregerson HG. (2006) Religious coping is associated with the quality of life of patients with advanced cancers. *Journal of Palliative Medicine* 9: 646–657.

Thombre A, Sherman AC and Simonton S. (2010) Religious coping and posttraumatic growth among family caregivers of cancer patient in India. *Journal of Psychosocial Oncology* 28: 173–188.

Utne I, Miaskowski M, Paul SM and Rustøen T. (2013) Association between hope and burden reported by family caregivers of patients with advanced cancer. *Supportive Care in Cancer* 21(9): 2527–2535.

Van Puymbroeck M, Hinojosa MS and Rittman MR. (2008) Influence of sense of coherence on caregiver burden and depressive symptoms at 12 months post stroke. *Topics in Stroke Rehabilitation* 15(3): 272–278.

Vilaythong AP, Arnau RC, Rosen DH and Mascaro N. (2003) Humor and hope: Can humor increase hope? *Humor* 16(1): 79–89.

Watson J. (2012) *Nursing. Human Caring Science*, 2nd ed. Boston, MA: Jones & Bartlett.

5

Impact of Caring on Families and Carers

Introduction

In the previous chapters, an overview of stress response and coping with the caregiving role has been presented, and several theories have been explored to help understand the underpinning process. The final component in the stress process is the signs of the impact on the caregiver's well-being and health. The aim of this chapter is to focus on the consequences of caregiving both as a negative and as a positive phenomenon, in an effort to provide a balanced understanding of the impact of caregiving on families and carers. The chapter begins with the adverse effects of caregiving and effects on the physical health of both caregivers and care recipients. This is followed by other negative consequences, including social isolation and emotional and psychological impact of caring, i.e., caregiver strain and burden, depression and loss and, finally, the impact on roles and relationships. The final section of the chapter explores the positive impact of caregiving, focusing on the conceptual issues of adversarial growth and post-traumatic growth (PTG) and finding meaning through caregiving.

Being a caregiver can be a highly stressful, complex and challenging experience, and the welfare of family caregivers is a major concern. This experience and associated stress process reflect a process that changes over time, i.e., over the carer's career. The manifestations of this process are the psychological and physical health and well-being of the carer. This impact is multidimensional and may affect family caregivers and family health differently depending on the unique caregiving situations, including objective elements such as the nature and time spent in carrying out caregiving tasks, for example, activities of daily living, and subjective elements such as emotional, social and relational stressors associated with the caregiving role.

Over the last two decades, the negative consequences of caregiving such as burden, depression, distress and stress have dominated the literature. Another way of viewing the negative consequences of caregiving is through the term 'suffering' or 'human cost', many of which are hidden from view. As articulated by Monin and Schulz (2010), suffering is a holistic construct defined by three dimensions: psychological, physical and existential. All three dimensions can be experienced by family caregivers, but it is important to note that these dimensions do not necessarily manifest as separate entities and may change during the course of a carer's career.

Understanding and assessing the negative impact of caregiving is essential if nurses are to implement appropriate interventions aimed at alleviating these potential negative consequences. In addition, a caregiver's health can determine the potential for the caregiver to continue providing care or the need to provide alternatives to family caregiving, such as respite care of residential/care homes. It is important that nurses understand not just the carer's experiences but what factors influence a carer's ability to provide effective care to their loved ones because caregiving has become a critical and major healthcare issue and a global healthcare resource. Furthermore, adverse consequences of caregiving may also inadvertently affect the care recipient. Equally important is the need to understand the positive effects so that these can be maximised to enhance the caregiver's well-being.

Physical Impact

Caregiving and Its Effect on Caregivers' Physical Health

The effects of caregiving on physical health have received less attention than the effects on psychological health. Yet the evidence suggests that caregiving can have a deleterious effect on the physical well-being of caregivers because caregiving often involves some level of physical effort. This physical work may include providing a wide variety of assistance with activities of daily living, including bathing, toileting, dressing, lifting moving and transferring, and doing additional physical chores. Prolonged activation of bodily systems is known to manifest in physical symptoms such as fatigue sleep and gastric disturbances. These important concepts provide a conceptual basis for quantifying the physiological effects of stress in carers. However, few caregiver studies have explored this link between high allostatic load and worsening physical health. In a study of older dementia caregivers, allostatic load score increased over a 2-year follow-up (Clark et al. 2007). Also, Roapke et al. (2011) found that Alzheimer's caregivers had significantly higher allostatic load compared to non-caregivers ($p < 0.05$) determined by a variety or both psychosocial and biological measures. In reality, measuring allostatic load (i.e. plasma cortisol and catecholamine levels and physiological parameters such as blood pressure and heart rate) may not be practical. More research in this area is needed to develop and validate sensitive, non-invasive and quantitative measures of allostatic load and to develop models that predict health outcomes.

Several reviews and two meta-analyses have found that informal caregivers have poorer physical health than non-caregivers (Pinquart and Sörensen 2003, 2006, 2007; Vitaliano et al. 2003). On the whole, these studies suggest that caregiving is associated with negative physical health consequences such as sleep disruption, fatigue, muscular injuries and aggravation of chronic diseases such as arthritis. In addition, these increased caregiver demands were associated with higher physical effect when caring for male and older caregivers and caregivers of people with dementia. Compared to non-caregivers, caregivers often experience psychological, behavioural and physiological effects that can contribute to impaired immune system function and coronary heart disease, and even early death. In a landmark prospective population-based cohort study, Schulz and Beach (1999) reported that stressed caregivers experienced 63% greater risk for mortality within 5 years when compared with to non-caregivers. The study concluded that caregiver stress was an independent risk factor for caregiver mortality. Other studies suggest that caregiving for a disabled or ill spouse was associated with increased risk of coronary heart disease (Lee et al. 2003).

A broad range of outcome measures have been studied, including cellular and organ-based physiological measures. These outcome measures have been linked to stressors such as the duration and type of caregiving along with other factors derived from caregivers interacting with others such as family conflict and role changes. Evidence does indicate that the nature of the relationship between the caregiver and the care recipient may play a key role in the degree of these outcomes. For example, duration of caregiving seems to have less effect on parental caregivers than spouse or adult children caregivers. Zehner Ourada and Walker (2014) conducted a survey of 293 American caregiving parents and caregiving adult children and found that caregiving parents have poorer self-rated health and more chronic health conditions than caregiving adult children. In addition, caregiving men are more likely to suffer physical ill heath than caregiving women (Pinquart and Sörensen 2006) and ethnic minority caregivers have poorer physical health than Caucasian caregivers (Pinquart and Sörensen 2005). Other caregiver characteristics correlate with physical health; for example, older caregivers are more at risk of worsening physical health than younger caregivers. Physical health outcomes many also be influenced by the intensity of caregiving and specific characteristics of the care recipient, such as night-time wandering or restlessness which may result in sleep deprivation, and a person's impulsive and violent behaviours can result in carers being directly injured.

Several assessment tools specifically designed to measure caregivers' physical well-being exist, for example, the Pittsburgh Sleep Quality Index. These tools can be easily administered to capture a more comprehensive view of the caregivers' quality of life in the domain of physical well-being. However, measuring physical well-being in caregivers in this way is not without its challenges, not least because caregivers are so focused on caring for their loved ones that they may be reluctant to declare their own healthcare needs. Neglecting their own health, by putting others before them, can manifest in many ways such as not attending outpatient appointments or skipping scheduled appointments with their general practitioner due to restriction on their time and poor dietary habits as a result of caregiving tasks. In addition, due to their busy daily activities, caregivers may forget to take prescriptions for their own chronic illnesses, which can result in poor control of their own conditions. New caregivers may also have to change their health-related activities such as diet and cessation of leisure time and exercise regimes which may negatively influence their health and well-being. Poor physical health not only places the caregiver at risk but can create potential negative risks to other family members and friends and the care recipient, as they are reliant on the ability of the carer to provide care, which in turn may result in difficulties in carers maintaining their caregiving responsibilities. Moreover, physical effort in caring, such as lifting and moving a loved one and other physical chores, can result in muscular back and shoulder strains or injury. It must be noted that for some caregivers increased physical activity can lead to health improvements.

Early recognition of and intervention for caregivers' physical strain is therefore important in preventing the onset of major health problems for caregivers and any adverse effect on their loved ones. Optimising the variables that may help to buffer the stress that is inevitably associated with sudden events such as family injury or illness should be a specific focus for nurses, especially when the patient is discharged from hospital or rehabilitation. Further research is required in this area in order to gain a better understanding of the factors that influence psychological and physiological responses to environmental stressors. However, if nurses recognise physiological effects of caring, there may be an opportunity for preventative healthcare.

Adverse Effects of Caregiving: Risk to Care Recipients

The demanding work of caregivers may put their loved ones at risk of harm. Although the care they carry out may have good intention, their lack of knowledge and skill may result in unintentional harm and inadvertently in hospitalisation, adding to the caregivers' stress. Caring for a spouse with significant cognitive or physical impairment may result in neglect or abusive behaviours, such as shouting. Unintentional neglect may also occur if a loved one is unable to communicate their needs due to cognitive or communication barriers, coupled with caregivers not being unable to understand or know how to deal with particular issues such as pain management and moving and handling their loved ones.

The importance of a carer's knowledge and skills is heightened when it comes to administering medications. Often, carers manage complex medication regimes without prior knowledge. The 'daily hassles' related to medication administration, e.g., frequent and complex medication regimes, what to do when a dose is missed or adjusting doses, not only are very time consuming but can increase stress and have a significant effect on the ability of the caregiver to carry out their responsibility. Little research exists on this subject, but Travis et al. (2000) found that caregivers manage between 1 and 14 medications on a daily basis and often miss doses due to their work schedules. Medication mismanagement is a common and well-recognised issue amongst the elderly. The caregiver who is responsible for the administration of medications also watches for signs of side effects; however, this requires a degree of health literacy, in other words, the carers' capacity to obtain, process and understand information in order to make appropriate decisions. Elderly caregivers with low health literacy are particularly at risk of making medication errors (e.g. dosing and misinterpretation of written instructions) which may result in adverse drug events and hospitalisation. By being aware of family carers who may be at risk of experiencing intense medication hassles, such as the elderly, nurses can target interventions to provide medication administration support. For example, targeted education on medication includes recognising adverse drug effects they may see as their family member's condition changes and what to do about it if they occur.

Key Points

- Caregivers are at serious risk for poor physical health outcomes.
- Physical stress of caregiving can affect the physical health of the caregiver.
- Poor physical health of a carer may place the care recipient at risk for harm.

Psychosocial Impact

Social Isolation

Most human beings seek company or relationships in their lives. This social engagement for many provides support, a sense of belonging and contributes to feelings of happiness and contentment. Belonging is a multidimensional construct of relatedness to persons, place and things and is critical to a person's social well-being (Hill 2006). But caring for someone can be the most socially isolating occupation even for those with a strong social network and is a key theme amongst caregivers. It has been studied by several disciplines ranging from psychology and social work to public health, and several definitions of social isolation can be found in the literature. One of the widely quoted definitions of social isolation was proposed by Nicholson (2009, p. 1346):

a state in which the individual lacks engagement with others, has a minimal
number of social contacts and they are deficient in fulfilling and quality
relationships.

Put simply, isolation is a lack of normal social contacts or social connectedness. The negative
health-related consequences of being socially isolated are well established and as a result have
attracted increasing interest from various authorities, including the UK government. For
example, the launch of national networks to support loneliness in older people such as the
Campaign to End Loneliness in 2011 and the more recent Care and Support White Paper
(DH 2012) recognises loneliness and social isolation as a major issue in society. According to
the World Health Organization (WHO 1948), health is defined as a state of complete physical,
mental and social well-being and not merely the absence of disease or infirmity. Thus, holistic
nursing care should include social well-being aspects which encompass isolation in order that
nurses can understand how it may affect caregivers and take steps to reduce it.

There is much debate on the distinction between social isolation and loneliness. The more
recent literature delineates social isolation into two categories: (1) subjective isolation, which
refers to the perceived isolation by the individual and feelings of isolation, separation from
others, and (2) objective isolation, which quantifies the level of isolation, such as the size of the
social network or amount of social support and the number of interactions with others. Both
are considered to be interlinked, each contributing to negative health effects. Loneliness can be
defined as a discrepancy between the individual's desired and actual social relations (Peplau
and Perlman 1982) and is often referred to as perceived social (subjective) isolation (Cacioppo
et al. 2014, 2015), in other words, is regarded as the psychological aspect of social isolation.
Loneliness has been the subject of considerable research most notably by the American
psychologist John T. Cacioppo and his colleagues. Cacioppo and colleagues' evolutionary
perspective of loneliness presents loneliness as a powerful adaptive signal, similar to hunger
and thirst, that motivates a person to alter their behaviour in a way that will increase survival.

According to Nicholson (2009), both loneliness and social isolation need to be viewed
as separate concepts, whereby social isolation may lead to loneliness but loneliness is not
a necessary condition of social isolation. Therefore, it is possible to be lonely even when a
carer is not isolated, for example, when their spouse is hospitalised or placed in a nursing
or residential home, and equally a carer may feel alone even though they are surrounded by
family or friends. Therefore, 'feeling alone' is not synonymous with 'being alone'. Perhaps
more importantly for caregivers, this implies that increasing social contact does not
necessarily mitigate against loneliness. Whilst illness, trauma or disability can be a singular
lonely experience for a patient, it can also be isolating for family caregivers, and a range
of circumstances, often imposed on them, may cause the caregiver to experience social
isolation. Social isolation can be influenced by three main contextual factors – individual
(caregiver's characteristics such as the ability or desire to go out and see others age),
community (access and availability of resources such as respite care, community support
groups and the environment that the carer lives in) and societal factors (governmental
policies that influence transportation networks and financial benefits).

Due to their caregiving demands exceeding their capacity to socially interact with others, a
caregiver's social life can be dramatically disrupted, reducing opportunities to maintain social
networks and engage in leisure and work activities. Lone caregivers may feel unsupported
by their family and friends, further compounding their sense of loneliness. Caregiving can
prevent carers from leaving their home as often as they used to and they may sacrifice their
leisure pursuits and hobbies and restrict time with friends and family, all resulting in families

and friends drifting away. If the carer has to give up or reduce employment to care, then this may impose financial restrictions that may prevent them from engaging in social activities that they did before, their world shrinks and they may express feelings of being 'under house arrest'. For caregivers who provide more long-term care, for example, when caring for a disabled child or elderly person, this may make getting out of the house problematic/difficult, due to the immense effort and planning required in doing so. This reduced contact with the community can lead to feelings of social alienation and isolation. Instead of the family home being a place of freedom, it can become more of a cage or prison. In addition, carers may feel invisible as the person they are caring for takes centre stage and the carer fades into the background. Caregivers, particularly those who care for people living with chronic illness, have also been identified in the literature as a group at risk of becoming isolated. For example, Drentea et al. (2006) found that caregivers of family members with Alzheimer's disease (AD) are particularly susceptible to isolation. Similarly, Braine (2011) found loneliness to be a key theme in caregivers of people with acquired brain injury (ABI). Age as a determinant of social isolation is not clear, partly due to the fact that most studies have been on older adults, thus giving a disproportionate view, although being an older carer is often associated with risks for social isolation such as limited mobility capacities and social networks.

An exemplar of environmental influence can be found in North West of England. According to the North West Public Health Observatory (2011), by 2033 the region of Cumbria has an ageing population with a prediction that 38.1% of the population will be over 60 years old compared to 28.2% in England. This area also has a reputation of attracting affluent older people seeking a better quality of life in the country side. This rural setting brings its own challenges for new carers who may have moved after retirement to a place that has limited access to immediate healthcare facilities and transportation services and who may be living away from other family members and friends, all contributing to the risk of social isolation and loneliness. In contrast, greater community networks create a sense of belonging and increase general health and well-being. Recognition by community nurses of carers residing in rural areas, with long distances between services, can significantly impact such a caregiver's loneliness and social isolation. Other influencing factors may need to be considered such as whether or not the caregiver lives with the person needing care and the severity of illness of the care recipient.

Substantial evidence demonstrates that social isolation and loneliness are associated with numerous negative health outcomes and a major risk factor for premature mortality (Cacioppo et al. 2015; Holt-Lunstad et al. 2015). Several meta-analysis and review papers have identified a long list of health conditions with which loneliness (subjective isolation) is associated, for example, depression, increased risk of coronary heart disease and stroke and diminished immunity and obesity, amongst others. In a meta-analysis by Holt-Lunstad and colleagues, the effects of social connection on health were comparable to smoking and about three times larger than obesity. Thus, social isolation and loneliness (subjective isolation) are major healthcare concerns for caregivers. Berkman et al. (2000) present a useful conceptual framework on how limited social networks impact negatively on health through three main pathways:

1. An increase in health-damaging behaviours such as alcohol consumption and smoking, being sedentary and neglecting their own health
2. Psychological behaviours such as decreased self-efficacy and sense of well-being and increased risk of depression and depressive symptoms
3. Physiological behaviours such as decreased immune response which can potentially lead to other health problems

Evidence suggests that social isolation in childhood, as a result of occupying isolating roles in their peer groups, can have a detrimental effect on their health in later life (Caspi et al. 2007). Nurses need to be mindful that for young carers this may be of particular importance as they may have to sacrifice their childhood activities to care. This may be due to lack of time available for them to socialise with their friends or the reluctance to do so due to their anxiety about the welfare of their parent they are caring for if they leave them to go out. They may even be reluctant to bring friends home. In a report by The Children's Society (2013), in England young carers are reported to be more likely to miss out on their school life as well as their social life, which affects their long-term education and employment prospects. This highlights the importance of looking at the life course of caregivers, as mentioned in Chapter 3.

Within the context of family and carers, it is critical that nurses capitalise on opportunities in the community to reduce caregiver's social isolation and loneliness to mitigate against potential adverse effects on their health and well-being. However, despite the substantial evidence linking social isolation with negative health outcomes, it is rarely assessed in the community setting. Understanding risk factors and associated variables of social isolation provides nurses with important areas to inquire about during their assessment of caregivers. One way of assessing contributing factors such as lack of belonging is to use appropriate rapid screening tools, although the number of instruments designed specifically to measure isolation is limited. The most commonly used instrument is the UCLA Loneliness Scale (Russell 1996) designed to assess subjective feelings of loneliness or social isolation and has been repeatedly validated, whereas the Lubben Social Network Scale (LSNS-6) (Lubben et al. 2006) is a popular measure of a person's social network or community.

Key Points

- Social isolation can be subdivided into subjective and objective isolation.
- Loneliness can be viewed as subjective social isolation.
- The quantity and quality of a carer's social relations are critical to the experience of social isolation.
- Loneliness and social isolation can have a severe detrimental effect on the health and well-being of a carer.

Caregiver Strain and Burden

One of the most studied areas of caregiving is the overall burden that the stress places on the family as a whole. Evidence suggests that there is considerable variation in how caregivers adapt to their caregiving demands, and the relation between caregiving and health is described generally in terms of stress. However, in the caregiving literature concepts, the terms burden, stress and strain are often used interchangeably, and in particular caregiver strain and burden are not always well conceptualised or well defined. To clarify, caregiver strain is usually referred to as the caregiver's perceived difficulty in performing their caregiving role and is termed 'role strain' (Archbold et al. 1990). The theory frequently applied to explain role strain is role theory, which posits the idea that humans act in varying and predictable ways based on expectations and conditions in social roles they assume (Brindle 1986). It is also argued that when individuals lack time and resources to fulfil the role expectations, role conflict and role overload occur. According to Goode (1960), role strain can be defined as the '…difficulty in meeting role demands' (p. 485). This is particularly relevant for caregivers as they assume the role of carer and at the same time hold multiple role obligations such as wife and daughter or husband and father, as well as employee and parent. Given that the roles that a carer undertakes are multifaceted, it should come as no surprise that role strain is not a singular concept and a number of dimensions have been identified along with scales to measure them.

The concept of caregiver 'burden' is one of the most commonly investigated caregiving outcomes. Interest in burden grew in the 1950s and 1960s, principally in families of mental ill-health patients, as home care for the mentally ill grew in popularity. This deinstitutionalisation* movement in countries such as the United Kingdom saw researchers aiming to explore the impact of behaviour of mentally ill people on families on families. American researchers Clausen and his colleagues reported on their earliest study in 1955 the consequences of mental illness on the family and were the first to use the term 'family burden' in their pioneering research that explored the impact of mental illness on spouses. These early findings were published in a series of papers in the *Journal of Social Issues*. A decade later, as home care increased in popularity, English psychiatrists Grad and Sainsbury (1963) noted the heavy responsibility and increased economic and emotional load borne by the families of the mentally ill and stated that burden was the negative impact on the family caused by caring for ill members. Subsequent years saw a growing interest and a multitude of definitions. To date, there is no singular or uniform conceptualisation or definition of caregiver burden in the literature and little consensus on how to measure it.

Despite its importance, the International Classification of Diseases (ICD-10) does not have a code for caregiver burden. This can, in part, be attributed to the fact that the concept has evolved from being viewed as a single construct to one that is multidimensional, e.g., subjective and objective burden. Zarit et al. (1980, p. 261) proposed a useful definition:

> the extent to which caregivers perceived their emotional, physical health, social life, and financial status as a result of caring for their relative.

This definition emphasises the multidimensional and negative consequences of caregiving. Caregiver burden can be defined as the overall consequences associated with a demanding and stressful caregiver situation or the load borne by the caring for a person who may be acutely or chronically ill or a dependent person (e.g. disabled or elderly family member). This may include any disruption in daily routine, social relationships and other activities that may occur as a result of caregiving. Put more simply, burden is the perceived stress or the perception that the situation exceeds a carer's available resources. The resources may come from the carer themselves or from external informal or formal support. It can be argued that some burdensome activities, such as household chores and routines, will occur in normal life. Therefore, caregivers might experience burden regardless of the presence or absence of caring for a family member. Although burden is a unique experience for each individual caregiver, it may be shouldered by a single or *primary caregiver* or distributed amongst several family members.

Although caregiving may result in massive savings for both families and governments alike, it may also result in increased costs financially to the caregiver as they often forgo the opportunity to be part of the labour market, for example, choosing part time over full time employment as a result of their competing caregiving demands on their time. Depending upon the family's socioeconomic status and other characteristics such as gender, this can have a considerable financial burden on society and increase caregiver risks for negative

---

* See care in the community in Chapter 2.

outcomes. As the United Nations (2013) states, by the end of the century, there will be seven times more people over the age of 80 than in 2013 worldwide and about a 51% fall in working age population by 2050, representing a significant increase in family, societal and healthcare burden.

Burden is commonly understood to have two distinct components – subjective and objective burden – which have added to the complexity of the concept. Hoeing and Hamilton (1966) were one of the first researchers to conceptualise burden into these two components. Subjective burden relates to the psychological consequences for the family and is defined as individuals' personal appraisals of the situation and the extent to which carers perceive the burden of care, i.e., the emotional or psychological reactions which caregivers experience such as feelings of loss and grief, anxiety and depression, stress of coping and frustration caused by changing relationships. Objective burden relates to the actual events and activities, physical or practical, experienced by family caregivers such as the disruption of family relationships; constraints in social, leisure and work activities; financial difficulties; number of hours involved in care provided; and negative impact on their own physical health. These two components often interact with each other and this emphasises the complex nature of caring. Some carers performing caregiving duties see them as part of their daily routine (e.g. assistance with activities of daily living), whereas others performing comparable duties perceive them as burdensome. Moreover, coping with the burden of caregiving may not necessarily be a negative experience, i.e., carers may be burdened whilst experiencing a sense of well-being. Though the literature is clear, burden on family caregivers leads to negative consequences not only for themselves but also for patients and other family members.

Assessment of Burden

Screening, assessing and monitoring levels of caregiver burden are crucial. Researchers have predominantly explored and measured caregiver burden by quantitative tools measuring both subjective and objective burden components. These tools are helpful for healthcare professionals in identifying those at risk for caregiver burden. Criticism has been levelled at this approach, despite their ease of use for several reasons: first, they fail to address the context issues surrounding caring, for example, cultural influences; second, it does not distinguish between the two components as they include both; and third, the measures do not encompass all aspects of the caregiver's burden experience. Montgomery et al. (1985) argues that a family may experience high levels of objective burden but low levels of subjective burden, or vice versa, and that different factors predict each type of burden. Recent studies have led to a more refined understanding of caregiver burden along with the identification of contributing and protecting factors. To reflect some of the advances in our understanding of burden and its multidimensional perspective, several burden subscales have been developed to include the measures of specific constructs such as strain; others have been developed to measure specifically the different components of burden, whereas some are more encompassing, such as the Zarit Burden Interview (ZBI) (Zarit et al. 1986). This tool is the most commonly used instrument in the literature and widely used across Europe and America; this was initially developed for use in caregivers of dementia patients but has since been used in a much broader context. Consisting of 22 items in its full version and 12 items in its short version, it measures objective and subjective burden as perceived by caregivers and has demonstrated high consistency and validity – the higher the score, the higher the burden. Although the tool was not originally developed for use in clinical practice, it does provide a good measure of the extent of caregiver burden. Many other caregiver burden scales exist, such as the Caregiver Burden Inventory, and several have been translated into other languages. Some measures of burden are one-dimensional, for example, the 13-item caregiver strain index (Robinson 1983), which measures strain related to care provision. This measure was developed for administrating 2 months of post-hospital discharge, and thus caution is required when applying it to different points in a carer's career. In addition, some scales are focused on specific diseases of the person being cared for. This has important implications for nurses working with family caregivers in that they need to be mindful of the context of research studies and applicability to their own clinical setting. Awareness of the different tools and what aspect of burden they are measuring deserves careful consideration, especially when identifying a burden screening tool in practice.

Thinking Box

Consider what might be happening psychologically, physically, financially and socially in a family that you have cared for.

Are these changes causing strain/burden and if so why?

How might this be identified?

Influencing Factors

It is crucial that factors that increase the risk or vulnerability for perceiving burden are understood as this will enable the nurse to target those who are at risk of burden and implement appropriate interventions to alleviate burden. There is a wealth of evidence that supports the notion that the characteristics of both the family caregiver and care recipient impact the caregiver's experience of burden. Of the caregiver characteristics, gender differences have been a prominent topic of interest, although research findings in this area are inconsistent. Overall, most studies suggest that women experience more burden and distress than men as caregivers, although some studies have found that men experience more burden and distress, whilst other studies found no gender differences (Miller and Cafasso 1992). It is often hypothesised that women suffer more consequences of caregiving due to their typical engagement in more personal care and hands-on care activities than men in the caregiver role, which makes them more vulnerable to the stressors of caregiving. Focused studies on caregivers of particular illnesses/diseases indicate that women traditionally bear the responsibility of caregiving across cultures. In the worldwide community-based epidemiological surveys, levels of burden across 19 countries were assessed in carers for first-degree relatives with chronic physical and mental health conditions (Viana et al. 2013). These researchers found women reported consistently significantly more burden than men with family caregiving demands and experienced greater subjective burden associated with caregiving. Equally, Shaley et al.'s (2013) cross-sectional community epidemiological surveys, which focused on older caregivers across 20 countries, reported that women reported significantly more burden than men. This may be attributed to the typical engagement in more personal care and hands-on care activities than men in the caregiver role. Notably, male caregiver experiences are conspicuously lacking from the literature. A carer's individual coping strategy and how these are used in mediating the stress associated with caregiving have also been found to be correlated with burden. Although the literature is limited and inconclusive in this area, avoidance coping and emotion-focused coping are positively associated with burden (Del-Pino-Casado et al. 2011).

Environmental factors have also been found to be influential, such as availability of social support and resources. Adelman et al. (2014) identify risk factors for caregiver burden, which include the following: being female, having low educational attainment, residing with the care recipient, depression, social isolation, financial stress, higher number of hours spent on caregiving and lack of choice in being a caregiver. In an American survey of caregiver burden, using a level of care index (number of hours of care given), high burden was most common in primary caregivers living with their loved ones and not employed whilst caregiving (National Alliance for Caregiving and AARP 2009). Similarly, Kim et al. (2012) examined the multidimensional predictors of caregiver burden in caregivers of persons with dementia and reported that increasing the number of hours devoted to caregiving was a significant predictor of caregiver burden.

The relationship of the caregiver to the person receiving care is also well established as an influencing factor. The literature consistently identifies the spouse at greatest risk of caregiver burden because they are more likely to live with the care recipient, have little choice in taking on the caregiving role and are more vulnerable because of their older age and associated morbidities (Burton et al. 1997; Conde-Sala et al. 2010; Shahly et al. 2013). In a meta-analysis by Pinquart and Sorensen (2011), although no difference in the overall level of burden between spouses and adult children was found, spouses reported higher levels of physical burden but not more emotional burden than adult child caregivers. In a cross-sectional worldwide survey in 19 countries, first-degree female relatives (spouse, parent and children) reported significantly more burden than men across a wide range of countries (Viana et al. 2013).

Diversity within society also makes this an important consideration in caregiver burden identification and assessment. Culture shapes our perceptions of family responsibilities and it is known that differing cultures may express differing levels of distress from caregiving. In an early review of 18 studies, Janevic and Connell (2001) found that Caucasian caregivers tend to report greater depression and appraised caregiving as more stressful than African-American caregivers. Other studies since then have identified that caregivers experience similar levels of caregiver burden but express them differently. European studies show that the ways in which family carers cope with their loved one and the burden imposed by the caring role are influenced by cultural factors (e.g. strength and value of family ties) which affect their appraisal of the situation, with major differences between Northern and Southern European countries (Novi et al. 2013). Other cultural differences are noteworthy; for example, amongst Asian families where traditional Confucian and Buddhist concepts dominate, there is a greater sense of responsibility for care of family members and a reluctance to involve others in caregiving. This may have significant influence on the caregiver's degree of burden and connects with notions of familism, as mentioned in Chapter 2.

Studies also indicate that there are variations in burden experiences between countries due to the levels of service provision. For example, in mental illness studies, care burden differences persist despite controlling for patient and caregiver characteristics, and this can be attributed to the differences in healthcare systems in the countries studied (Van Wijngaarden et al. 2003; Roick et al. 2007; Carra et al. 2012). These studies draw attention to the different contextual factors associated with belief systems about mental health, mental health service provisions and welfare systems cross-culturally. It appears that both culture and demographic factors are key influences in determining the degree of perceived family caregiver burden.

Although burden is a unique experience for each individual caregiver, specific care recipient factors have been found to facilitate the prediction of burden in family members, for example, greater severity of illness and symptoms and longer duration of illness (e.g. schizophrenia and neurodegenerative diseases). As far back as the 1970s, studies carried out on caregivers of people with traumatic brain injury (TBI) have reported that cognitive and behavioural disturbances in the injured individual are more important than the physical injury in predicting the levels of burden experienced by family members. Research literature on burden has extensively been studied in four main caregiver population groups – caregivers of dementia, mental illness, cancer and ABI. This does not indicate that other population groups receiving less attention suffer less caregiver burden; in fact some diseases may result in more caregiver burden than others. Several examples of this can be drawn from the literature. The unpredictability of multiple sclerosis (MS) can affect the caregiver in a way unlike other chronic diseases as caregivers are unable to predict the onset of a relapse, the progression of the disease or even the functional ability of the patient over the course of a day (McKeown et al. 2004). This is compounded by the fact that it is not just the physical symptoms that increase with time, increasing the caregiver burden, but also the psychological and emotional aspects of MS that present significant challenges for family caregivers.

As mentioned earlier, one of the earliest investigations of caregiving and family burden focused on the consequences of discharging the mentally ill from institutions and placing them in relatives' homes (Montgomery et al. 1985). Since deinstitutionalisation, caregivers have increasingly assumed greater responsibility for the care of their mentally ill relatives in the community, and several studies suggest that higher burden is associated with mental illness than physical conditions (Hastrup et al. 2011; Pinquart and Sorensen 2011; Viana et al. 2013). When comparing families of patients with schizophrenia with long-term physical disease such as brain disease, diabetes, chronic heart and kidney disease, Magliano et al. (2007) found objective burden to be higher in brain diseases and subjective burden to be higher in schizophrenia and brain diseases compared to the other groups. It is also worth noting here that according to various reports from the World Health Organization, mental illness and neurological conditions are the leading causes of disease burden worldwide, in particular neurological disorders are one of the greatest threats to public health (Mathers and Loncar 2007; Murray et al. 2010). Given these facts, caregiver burden has the potential to be a significant problem worldwide especially amongst carers of people with neurological diseases.

There are clearly many influencing factors, but it is beyond the scope of this book to explore them in more detail, but what is clear is that caregiving burden extends across a range of mental and physical conditions, health delivery systems and cultures. Recognising the primary disease of the care recipient can facilitate predictions of caregiving burden. More research is required to illuminate the impact of different illnesses in different cultures on family burden, especially as we live in a global society. Moreover, understanding the effects of different diseases on carer burden will enable the nurse to target assessment and tailor appropriate services and interventions that may help to alleviate carers' burden and improve the quality of life for both caregiver and care recipient.

Failure to identify families' and carers' ability to cope in their caregiving role can lead to carer burden with serious consequences for the health of both carer and care recipient. Besides understanding care recipients' disease or illness, carers need to be able to cope with problems and feelings that continued caring triggers. The lack of proper preparation to deal with these situations can lead to different levels of burden and increased burden as the patient's condition deteriorates. Therefore, efforts to identify, assess, reduce and monitor caregiver burden are important healthcare issues. It is important that our understanding of burden continues to be refined so that healthcare professionals can target those caregivers who are at increased risk or burden and develop and implement effective interventions so that caregiving is not compromised.

Key Points

- Caregiver burden and strain are difficult to conceptualise.
- Caregiver burden is multidimensional.
- Stress theories underpin subjective and objective burden.
- Caregiver strain and burden result in elevated stress amongst carers, which can result in serious health consequences.

Depression

Depression amongst caregivers is well documented, with a consistently high level of depressive symptoms reported when compared to non-caregivers. For example, Zarit (2006) reports clinically significant depression in 40%–70% of caregivers with approximately a quarter to one-half of these carers meeting the DSM-IV criteria for depression. Studies showed that middle-aged and older women who provided care for an ill spouse or a spouse with disability were almost six times as likely to have depressive or anxious symptoms as were those who had no caregiving responsibilities (World Federation of Mental Health 2010). However, most of the literature in this area is focused on caregivers of people with dementia. The few studies available in other caregiver groups also point to consistently higher rates of depression than non-caregivers and the general population, for example, stroke (Denno et al. 2013) and TBI (Ennis et al. 2013). This may well be due to the intensity of the caregiving (e.g. time involved in caregiving and level of physical tasks) and reduced social contact.

Caregiver depression studies have also focused on how caregiver burden may lead caregivers to being more vulnerable to depression. As the care recipient's condition worsens and the intensity of the caregiving increases, so does the level of depressive symptoms of the caregiver (Mohamed et al. 2010; Denno et al. 2013). The impact of caregiver depression is further complicated by its association with physical health, i.e., as the health of the caregiver declines, their depressive symptom increases (Smith et al. 2011). This raises the importance of reassessing caregivers as their health may decline over time, necessitating a need for more assistance in their caregiving responsibilities and thus helping to prevent the onset of depression. Moreover, problematic psychological and cognitive symptoms that are often exhibited in a range of patient groups such as dementia and ABI have been found to be a predictor of caregiver depressive symptoms. Other factors associated with caregiver depression are worthy of note and include poor-quality relationship between the caregiver and the care recipient, caregivers' previous physical and mental health status, gender, and lack of availability of social support.

Caregivers who have a significantly depressed mood may be adversely affected in their ability to perform caregiving tasks, observe and thus identify care needs of their loved one, which may result in neglect. The caregiving literature clearly indicates that the relationship between depression, burden and grief is complex, but each needs to be considered as a separate entity. Further research that describes influencing factors and the characteristics of caregivers who are most at risk for depressive symptoms is warranted in order to identify early those in need of intervention.

Loss and Grief Associated with Caregiving

Introduction

In general, we connect loss and the associated grief with the death of a loved one; however, family caregivers' experience losses that are much more complex and broader than this. They may be confronted with a multitude of losses which often are unspoken and are experienced privately during their caring career. This section aims to illuminate these losses and some of the theoretical perspectives in relation to loss and grief so that nurses can identify and understand caregiving experiences of loss in order to support and offer help. Caregiving is fraught with challenges, uncertainties and losses, and grief accompanies many carers in their caring journey. By understanding the complexity of loss in relation to caregiving, nurses can provide more sensitive care and help families and caregivers develop a therapeutic response to loss and grief. Working with and recognising grief and loss issues, which may manifest in many different forms and guises, is an important part of nursing care. However, the exploration and application of grief and loss theory from a perspective other than death has received relatively little attention in the nursing literature.

Several terms are commonly associated with loss, i.e., bereavement, mourning and grief. Bereavement can be defined as the objective reality of facing the loss of an important person, whereas grief is the subjective response to the loss (bereavement). Mourning, however, refers to the social manifestation of grief, i.e., the public display of grief, and is influenced by personal and religious beliefs and culture. Grief is a universal, natural, subjective human experience and commonly associated with death, but also with other losses.

The grief of caregivers is complex and often greater in intensity than the grief experienced after the death. In many cases, loss is a constant companion to illness, for patients and their families and caregivers. The multiple losses that family caregivers may experience may be very apparent such as loss of life, future and freedom, whilst others are more subtle such as loss of hopes, dreams and aspirations and expectations that they had for their loved ones and themselves (Braine 2010). Family caregivers may also experience losses related to varying aspects of the person they are caring for, including loss of a reciprocal relationship and companionship, shared goals, mutual support and family roles. Losses may also permeate other aspects of their everyday lives with a loss of freedom, inability to pursue leisure activities and perceived loss of normality in their everyday lives (Braine 2011). For many caregivers, a loss or disrupted sense of normality (i.e. routine and rhythm in everyday activities) may be evident by the loss of simple pleasures in life such as having private time for oneself or eating meals together as a family.

Given that prolonged illness trajectories often characterise chronic illness today, caregivers' losses may extend over several years, for example, in the case of dementia or ABI. During difficult periods, such as changes in a loved one's behaviour or during a rapid decline in condition, family caregivers' sense of loss may even be intensified. For example, embarrassed by the behaviours of their loved ones and fear of public humiliation, some carers, restrict or curtail their public activities (Braine 2010).

Despite the prolific literature on grief in response to death, relatively little is known about the grief associated with the losses in regard to caregiving. Research began in this area in the late 1980s focusing particularly on dementia caregivers due to the gradual decline or death of a person with dementia. Dementia researchers in particular have focused on defining pre-death grief and exploring its impact on stress and depression with evidence suggesting that grief increases as dementia advances. Pauline Boss (1999) was one of the first researchers to theoretically examine the feelings of grief and loss associated with AD and coined the term 'ambiguous loss'. Parallel to this was the growing interest in family caregivers of people with TBI, which began in the 1970s. Lezak (1978) is one of the first investigators to emphasise the particular difficulties of a spouse caring for a person with TBI, who was not the same person pre-injury, as someone who 'lives in a social limbo' and '...cannot mourn decently' (Lezak 1978, p. 593). Later, the recurring, lingering and disjointed process of grieving of families following TBI was referred to as 'mobile mourning', and the term 'partial death' was used to describe the sense of loss that family members may experience (Muir and Haffey 1984).

The losses that caregivers may suffer and feel can provoke a significant grief reaction and is often an overlooked experience of the caregiver. Furthermore, the grief experienced as a result of these losses is often disenfranchised or unrecognised as they continue with their caregiving demands. Meuser et al. (2004) suggest that grief reaction to the many losses that caregivers face may be an essential factor that is related to, but potentially distinct from, the symptoms of stress. Varying terms have been used related to loss, grief and grief responses, such as pre-death grief, carer grief, chronic grief, anticipatory mourning, anticipatory grief and disenfranchised grief, which has led to considerable confusion and controversy in the literature. To complicate this further, Bruce and Schultz (2001) add the term 'non-finite loss', and Doka (2002) uses the term 'disenfranchised loss'. Arguably, all refer to pre-death grief, which begins with diagnosis and continues until physical death of the family member.

It is important to note before we discuss grief and loss in more detail that a caregiver's grief reactions and depression often present with very similar symptoms and behavioural manifestations. Whilst most of the literature on caregiver depression discussed earlier has tended to focus on depression from a burden and stress perspective, most have not taken into consideration that there is evidence to suggest an overlap between the two symptomatically and that some caregivers may not be depressed but are grieving (Walker and Pomeroy 1996; Sanders and Adam 2005).

In some circumstances, grief and multiple losses felt by caregivers may result in a complex condition as prolonged grief disorder (Prigerson et al. 2009) or sometimes as complicated grief. In their studies on caregivers of patients with disorders of consciousness, i.e., minimally conscious state (MCS) and vegetative state (VS), several Italian researchers reported significant levels of prolonged grief disorder (Chiambretto et al. 2010; Leonardi et al. 2012). Whilst the majority of these patients were located in institutions, caregiver's grief of patients in VS or MCS can be significant, and they should receive targeted support.

Pre-Death Grief

Within the caregiving literature, there is little consensus and confusion on pre-death grief as the concept is often used interchangeably with others as mentioned earlier. In an attempt to analyse the concept of pre-death grief, Lindaer and Harvath (2014) concluded that there is evidence of a distinction between pre-death grief, chronic sorrow and anticipatory grief. The researchers concluded that pre-death grief in the context of dementia caregivers can be defined as the 'emotional and physical responses to the previewed losses in a valued care recipient' (p. 2303). The concept has been poorly studied, although in the dementia literature, there is a small growing body of evidence to suggest significant pre-death grief associated with caregiving (Sanders et al. 2008; Noyes et al. 2010). Marwit and Meuser (2005) posit that the grief of caregivers of persons with dementia is 'more akin to true grief [post-death grief] than it is to the anticipatory grief experienced by caregivers of patients with other terminal illness' (p. 202). This unique phenomenon of grieving the loss of the care recipient prior to the actual death and then grieving the loss of the person when the person actually dies has been referred to as 'dual dying' (Jones and Martinson 1992). In other caregiver populations, pre-death grief has received some attention. Marwit et al. (2008) assessed pre-grief death in cancer caregivers using the Marwit and Meuser caregiver grief inventory (MM-CGI). Carter et al. (2012) reported that pre-death grief was a significant finding in caregivers of Parkinson's disease and was significantly higher in those relatives whose loved ones had more severe symptoms. These studies indicate that pre-death grief exists in other caregiver populations, but further research is warranted to determine the presence and magnitude of pre-death grief in other caregivers.

Anticipatory Grief

There has been much debate and controversy over the concept and definitions of anticipatory grief. Erich Lindemann (1944) introduced the term 'anticipatory grief' in the 1940s when he focused on grief that a person might experience when the loss of a close loved one was anticipated but had not yet occurred. Some 40 years later, Theresa Rando (1986) expanded the definition of anticipatory grief and asserted that it is a response to a known terminal illness and that the full breadth of grief cannot be appreciated until the dying person is dead. Anticipatory grief refers to a grief reaction that occurs in anticipation of an impending loss, i.e. before the death of a loved one. For family caregivers, anticipatory grief is related to the actual and anticipated loss of the loved one's personhood and of their relationship with their loved one (Rando 1986). The definition of anticipatory grief offered by Rando (2000, p. 29) is widely accepted:

> The mourning, coping, interaction, planning, and psychological reorganisation that are stimulated and begun in part in response to the impending loss of a loved one and the recognition of associated losses in the past, present, and future.

More recently, debates suggest that this definition should be broader, involving those who are dying. Corr et al. (1997), however, point out that it is important to dispel the belief that the amount of grief experienced in anticipation of loss will decrease the remaining grief that is to be experienced after death. According to Rando (1986), anticipatory grief is a multidimensional construct consisting of emotions such as anger, guilt, anxiety, irritability, sadness, feelings of loss and decreased ability to function.

Despite the longevity of the term, anticipatory grief has been the subject of few studies. Rabin (1984), one of the first researchers on this topic in dementia care, wrote that many family caregivers of dementia go through a process called chronic grief. Since then a small growing number of studies have addressed this topic, although most have been amongst family caregivers of patients with dementia. Research suggests that family caregivers of people with dementia may experience grief prior to the death of their care recipients, partly due to the progression of multiple losses they experience and the chronic nature of caregiving. Furthermore, for these caregivers, losses will increase with time as the disease progresses, and they watch the gradual death of their loved one. This focus of anticipatory grief research in dementia perhaps relates to the unique issues that arise from dementia, i.e., the progressive deterioration of both cognitive and physical abilities, suggesting that caring for these patients is different from other patient populations. More recently, in dementia caregivers, Blandin and Pepin (2015) refer to this grief as a specific type of anticipatory grief called 'dementia grief'. This progressive cognitive decline that precedes physical decline and death in dementia has been referred to as a series of 'mini deaths' (Marwit and Meuser 2005). Given the nature of AD, caregivers are likely to experience numerous mini deaths and these experiences are likely to go unrecognised. A main research that focused on family caregivers of AD examined anticipatory grief between 3 and 6 years on average. Whether such grief is manifested early in the disease trajectory, i.e., at diagnosis, is unknown. Dementia caregivers surveys indicate that anticipatory grief may be as high as 71% (Diwan et al. 2009); more recently in a systematic review, Chan et al. (2013) reported rates between 47% and 71% and identified several factors that may increase anticipatory grief in dementia carers – carer depression, moderate to severe dementia and institutionalisation. Interestingly, anticipatory grief has also been found amongst family caregivers of persons with mild cognitive deficits, well before they meet the criteria for dementia (Garard et al. 2012; Fowler et al. 2013). Not only does this highlight a wider caregiver population that may experience anticipatory grief, but it also opens up the notion that other conditions and disease processes that feature cognitive impairment may result in anticipatory grief in caregivers, for example, ABI. A number of studies have suggested that anticipatory grief amongst caregivers can negatively influence their mood, physical health, productivity and social relationships and reduce their problem-solving abilities (Fowler et al. 2013), which is an important contributing factor in caregiver burden (Holley and Mast 2009).

Although the prevalence of anticipatory grief within other caregiver populations is largely unknown, a small body of evidence does suggest that this is an important consideration in family caregivers in a variety of contexts such as amyotrophic lateral sclerosis and MS (Grimby et al. 2015), chronic illnesses such as HIV and AIDS (Walker et al. 1996), Parkinson's disease (Johansson and Grimby 2014) and cancer (Johansson and Grimby 2012). Anticipatory grief has also been reported in parents of premature neonates, and most notable is that this reaction did not differ between the mother and father (Valizadeh et al. 2013). Similarly, Zamanzadeh et al.'s (2013) study revealed that fathers experience anticipatory grief reactions after the birth and hospitalisation of a premature infant. Both these recent studies stress that nurses and midwives should know the importance of recognising fathers' experiences and their grief reaction. Previous research in this area indicates that the grieving and mourning of mothers following the birth of their premature infant impair their ability to provide surveillance and maternal care in times of crisis and caused damage to the relationship between the mother and infant (Nyström et al. 2001).

In childhood studies, whilst much attention has focused on the process of actual bereavement and the needs of the family at this time, very few studies have addressed the parental ongoing losses as a result of their child's chronic illness. Childhood cancers, the most common cause of illness in children, can have a devastating psychosocial impact on the family with high degrees of distress and anxiety resulting from the uncertainty of the disease progression along with the loss of dreams and hopes for their child's future. A study by Beltrao et al. (2007) that explored maternal feeling when childhood cancer was diagnosed revealed intense feelings of pain, shock, sadness and despair.

Given that grief appears to be a key feature in many caregivers' experience, quantifying it is a necessary precursor to implementing grief-targeted interventions. Although there are a number of validated measures of grief, very few instruments have been developed to measure caregiver anticipatory grief. The two most commonly used instruments include the anticipatory grief scale (Theut et al. 1991), a 27-item scale originally validated on women spouse caregivers of AD patients representing thoughts, feelings and behaviours associated with the anticipation of the death of a spouse, and the MM-CGI

(Marwit and Meuser 2002), a 50-item self-report inventory designed specifically to measure grief in caregivers of dementia patients, which evaluates three areas of loss – personal sacrifice and burden (i.e. losses of time, freedom, sleep, health), worry and felt isolation (i.e. loss of personal connection to others and worries about the future) and heartfelt sadness and longing (i.e. emotional response to loss of relationship). Marwitt and Kay (2006) investigated the applicability of the MM-CGI in caregivers of ABI arguing that at the time there was no established inventory to measure grief in this caregiver's population. The researchers reported a similar result regarding caregivers of dementia people and argued that a slightly modified MM-CGI was reliable and valid. The inventory has also been subjected to further testing and validation on parent caregivers. First, Al-Gamal et al. (2009) developed and tested the MM-CGI Childhood Cancer to provide a suitable instrument to measure anticipatory grief in parents living with a child with cancer, and later Al-Gamal and Long (2013) took this a step further to establish a modified version of the MM-CGI Childhood Cancer to assess grief in parents of children with cerebral palsy. Both studies indicated a high prevalence of anticipatory grief, highlighting the growing need to recognise this important experience.

Anticipatory grief appears to be common in many caregiving groups. On this basis alone, nurses should anticipate and expect anticipatory grief in many caregivers and that they may need support. Given the increasing number of people living with chronic and terminal illness, due to medical advances and the ageing population, further research is required to illuminate the number of families experiencing anticipatory grief. Using a screening tool, such as the short version of the MM-CGI, will help in identifying caregivers with high levels of grief who may be in need of additional support and professional help.

Key Points

- Grief is a normal psychological and emotional response to significant loss.
- Anticipatory grief is an under-researched yet an important aspect of caregiving.
- Anticipatory grief is a phenomenon that describes the experience of the impending loss of a loved one.
- Studies indicate that caregivers experience significant pre-death losses and grief.
- Emerging evidence supports the notion of *dementia grief.*

Non-Finite Loss

Non-finite loss is continuous and insidious as the person gradually discovers the impact of a diagnosis, illness or other loss events. Bruce and Schultz (2001) developed the concept of non-finite loss to describe the lifespan of the grief felt by those family members who care for a child with developmental disabilities. The authors recognised that the parents experienced a continuous loss and grief that deny the families all of hopes, dreams and expectations as the child's disability unfolds through their lifespan. The authors distinguish *non-finite loss*, including disability, chronic and degenerative illness, from bereavement types of loss. This loss is often not identified or recognised and involves awareness of the discrepancy between life events and *what should have been*. Non-finite loss is continuous and insidious as the person gradually discovers the impact of a diagnosis, illness or other loss events (Bruce and Schultz 2001). Each loss experience is unique to the person (Rando 2000) and cannot be generalised or categorised. Arguably, the constant continuing presence of loss that is characteristic of degenerative diseases such as AD, MS and motor neuron disease can be captured by the term 'non-finite loss'.

Disenfranchised Grief

The societal context in which grief occurs also plays a crucial role in how a person experiences loss. Kenneth Doka's (1989) concept of disenfranchised grief draws attention to the ways in which the circumstances surrounding family members are outside the *grieving rules*. Doka (1989) defines disenfranchised grief 'as the grief that persons experience when they incur a loss that is not or cannot be openly acknowledged, publicly mourned, or socially supported' (p. 4). In other words, family members are disenfranchised from their grief, as society does not socially validate their pain. Doka (1989) identified three main reasons why disenfranchised grief can happen: (1) relationships are disenfranchised, i.e. not recognised; (2) losses are not recognised; and (3) grievers are not recognised. Disenfranchised grief is thus hidden grief because of the lack of social recognition. It may lay hidden for years, for example, the psychological death of a person with AD or following TBI. Disenfranchised grief is also particularly relevant for families in which relationships are not recognised such as friends or the *invisible family*, ex-spouses and young carers, although they may play an important part in caregiving. In addition, there may be family members that receive little or no social recognition of their perceived sense of loss of what they hoped or planned for or was never realized, such as young family caregivers and those caring for family members with learning disabilities. This type of grief may be difficult for caregivers to cope with as they may feel guilty for feelings that others may not agree with or understand.

Caregivers are hidden grievers and they often suffer in silence without the normal societal support. This failure to acknowledge another's loss according to Hardy and Laszloffy (2005) is to deny that person's humanity. It fails to respect the person's right to grieve and denies them the support and comfort they deserve. What Doka's work acknowledges is the importance of external factors on a person's experiences of loss and grief and raises the need for nurses to appreciate and support these hidden grievers.

Ambiguous Loss

Ambiguous loss is another theory which helps nurses to understand the social construction of an individual's grief experience. It is also helpful in understanding the grief experiences of families and caregivers. Research on ambiguous loss began in the 1970s with families of soldiers missing in action in Vietnam and Southeast Asia. Pauline Boss, an American family therapist, developed an understanding of ambiguous loss by observing families who had experienced this type of loss and described it as an unfinished loss as it defies closure until the person dies. The theory of ambiguous loss (Boss 1999, 2006) arose out of family stress theory, which posits that stress results whenever there is change within a family. According to Boss (1999), the most severe stressors are those changes that are not clear-cut but are ambiguous.

Although the death of a family member is a stressful event, it is validated through sociocultural processes that allow families to move forward through their grief. Conversely, when a family member disappears, for example, due to a debilitating illness (psychological loss), the remaining family members are thrown into uncertainty. This lack of verification of the loss generates a situation called ambiguous loss, i.e., the stressor/event or the A factor in the ABCX stress theory (see Chapter 3). There is no validation of loss (as with death); this loss is unclear loss and thus is without closure. Ambiguous loss is caused by external forces such as illness or injury which prevents clarity about a loved one's status as present or absent. Boss (1999, 2006) argues that this type of loss is traumatic and is *the most stressful kind of loss*. In relation to the stress process (see Chapter 3), not all stressors are clear-cut, and as a result ambiguity arises. In relating back to the ABCX stress theory, this perceived ambiguity (the C factor) arises out of the incongruence between physically presence and psychologically/ emotionally presence/absence. The premise of Boss's ambiguous loss theory is that ambiguity together with loss creates a powerful barrier to coping and grieving. When people experience ambiguous loss, they have difficulty making decisions, are unable to alter family roles and routines, question their beliefs and competence and become exhausted (Boss 1999, 2004, 2006). Boss argues that it is the ambiguity of the situation and not the psychological characteristics of the individual that contributes to perceptions of stress and inadequate functioning (Boss 1999, 2006), i.e., the outcome crisis (X factor). Families may find it impossible to work through their grief as they have been unable to renegotiate their new social boundaries. According to Boss (2006), in these uncharted territories, a family may become paralysed, unable to grieve and heal. It is the ambiguity of not knowing if a person is present or not that creates a complicated grief for family caregivers. The ambiguity surrounding this type of loss is so complex that Boss and Yeats (2014) state that a person's grief can be immobilised, thus freezing their grief. Ambiguity can lead to a blocked family system or to one that is in limbo, hindering the caregiving process. With no clear understanding of the situation, i.e., who does what in the family, mastering the situation is difficult.

Boss conceptualised two different types of ambiguous loss. The first type (type I) refers to a person who is physically absent but psychologically present in the family, which Boss refers to as 'leaving without saying goodbye'. This may refer to a family member who is absent physically, such as a missing child, or a family member being placed in a nursing or residential home. The second type (type II) refers to a person who is physically present and psychologically absent, for example, a cognitively and emotionally impaired person, such as in the case of dementia, brain injury, disorders of consciousness (e.g. coma) and certain mental illnesses, which boos refers to as 'goodbye without leaving'. No matter the situation, an ambiguous loss is one that is unclear, traumatic, externally caused, confusing and incomprehensible (Boss 2010).

Thinking Box

Can you think of some losses that often are experienced as ambiguous loss?

What might the effect be of *pile-up* of ambiguous losses?

Some, if not all, of these undoubtedly are applicable to many family caregiver's situations. When the role and identity of a family member are in question, for example, following injury or chronic illness, the family system is thrown into disarray and ambiguity thrives. Whilst this disruption can provide an opportunity for positive change, when the disruption is sudden, visually not apparent, misunderstood and undiagnosed, it can have negative consequences. Pauline Boss (1977), whilst working at the Naval Health Research Centre in the United States, introduced the view that boundary ambiguity was a major stressor based on families of the missing. Boss (1987, p. 709) defined family boundary ambiguity as

> ...a state when family members are uncertain in their perception of who is in or out of the family or who is performing what roles and task within the family system.

This uncertainty is thought to be a cause of high levels of stress and family dysfunction (Boss and Greenberg 1984). Boss (1999) contends that the higher the boundary ambiguity in the family system, the higher the family stress and the greater the individual and family dysfunction. Based on family systems theory (Chapter 2), family boundary ambiguity is defined as family not knowing who is in and who is out of the family system

(Boss and Greenberg 1984). Boundary ambiguity can result from two situations: (1) from outside the family when there is a lack of facts and certainty about the loss and (2) from inside the family when the perception of the events creates ambiguity by ignoring or denying the available facts. Thus, boundary ambiguity is likely to occur when family members experience a loss of someone within the family and have difficulty adjusting their perceptions surrounding the loss. When there is a perceptual difference between who is present physically and who is present psychologically, family ambiguity results. In Table 5.1, we can see the relationship between boundary ambiguity and ambiguous loss. Boundary ambiguity is conceived to be a continuous variable, because no family boundaries are clear at all times. The degree of ambiguity has been subjected to a scaled measurement such as the boundary ambiguity scale (the higher the score, the higher the ambiguity); however, this has rarely been applied in practice. The longer the boundary ambiguity, the greater the risk for stress; this has particular significance for families of ABI as the ambiguity may last for several years.

Ambiguous loss has been extensively documented in family stress research to explain the effect of family changes on family functioning, but within the healthcare literature, it has received relatively little attention. The ambiguous loss experienced by many caregivers is often not recognised, acknowledged or understood by either the caregiver themselves or by other family members and friends. Often, it is difficult for family members to admit that they feel a sense of loss because the person is still there and they believe they should feel grateful for this. This is particularly pertinent in the field of ABI when a family member suffers a road traffic injury and the family initially is thankful for their loved one surviving, despite the many losses they will experience as the impact unfolds over time.

Ambiguous loss is an under-researched aspect of loss, and there are very few published examples in the healthcare literature. Furthermore, in the main, ambiguous loss has been applied to families with adult members who are either physically or psychologically absent, which is echoed in the caregiving literature. In the case of caregiving, type II ambiguous loss has been studied in adult caregivers of families of AD (Garwick et al. 1994; Kaplan and Boss 1999), mild cognitive impairment (Blieszner et al. 2007), dementia (Dupuis 2002) and mental illness (Jones 2002), following brain injury and those who are in the ICU setting (Kean 2010), TBI (Laudau and Hissett 2008) and disorders of consciousness (Giovannetti et al. 2014). Dupuis (2002) found that ambiguous loss occurs even when the family member has been placed in residential care. Studies also indicate that ambiguous loss can help to understand parental losses as parents struggle with uncertainties of a sick

Table 5.1 Boundary ambiguity and ambiguous loss

High boundary ambiguity		Low boundary ambiguity	
Ambiguous loss type I	Ambiguous loss type II	No ambiguous loss	Clear-cut loss
Physically absent but psychologically present with *high* boundary ambiguity.	Physically present but psychologically absent with *high* boundary ambiguity.	Family members are both physically and psychologically present with clearer boundaries.	A family member is both physically and psychologically absent (i.e. death) with clearer boundaries.

or disabled child, although this is in very small, diverse populations, including parents of children with autism spectrum disorders (O'Brien 2007), parents of infants born prematurely (Golash and Powell 2003) and parents who had raised a child with profound disabilities and placed them in residential care (Roper and Jackson 2007). Mu et al.'s (2005) study on Taiwanese mothers of children with epilepsy found that high degrees of boundary ambiguity was positively correlated with depression. These studies stress the pervasiveness and longevity of ambiguous loss in diverse family caregivers but that it can have negative consequences on individual family members and the family as a whole. Despite there being no closure or resolution to ambiguous loss, recognition and labelling loss experience and providing information are important first steps that nurses can do to help these family members manage their loss. Both ambiguous loss and boundary ambiguity are intensely complex, but both offer a means of understanding traumatic family loss, although more research is needed.

Key Points

- Grief in caregivers is multidimensional.
- Both disenfranchised and ambiguous losses are important to bear in mind when caring for family members.
- Ambiguity about whether someone is present or absent can have negative health and well-being consequences.
- Caregivers experience multiple and cumulative losses.

Chronic Sorrow

Many people live with chronic illness and disability worldwide. In the United Kingdom, there are 12.2 million disabled people (long-standing illness, disability or infirmity), accounting for 19% of the population (Blackburn et al. 2010). In trying to cope with the ramification of caring for a loved one with a disability or chronic illness, some family members develop an emotional state known as chronic sorrow. Chronic sorrow, a type of identified grieving but distinctly different from bereavement and mourning, refers to a state of continually living with the loss of a loved one. The term was first introduced in 1962 by a rehabilitation counsellor, Simon Olshansky, based on his interviews with parents of children born with developmental disabilities. He described the normal, pervasive grief response associated with the suffering of parents dealing with mental disabled children as 'chronic sorrow', and theorized that this response would persist for the parents throughout the lifetime of their child (Olshansky 1962). This emotional response to an initial tragedy has also been described as an ongoing, living loss that is permanent, pervasive, recurring and cyclical in nature. Olshansky's definition was then later borne out in four studies conducted in the 1980s (Wikler et al. 1981; Fraley 1986; Burke et al. 1989; Damrosch and Perry 1989). All these studies carried out on families of mentally or physically disabled children provided evidence of chronic sorrow. Susan Roos (2002) argues that chronic sorrow is a normal response to living with irremovable loss.

Although varying definitions can be found concerning chronic sorrow, e.g., cyclic sadness, grief-relief process and living loss (Roos 1994), all are consistent in identifying the emotional experiences and the pervasive sense of loss. The defining characteristics include feelings that continue unabated, varying in intensity and occur periodically, and the family caregiver may experience feelings of anger, disbelief, disappointment, frustration, fear, helplessness, hopelessness, loneliness, loss and low self-esteem (Wilkinson 2000).

Following Olshansky's work, Copley and Bodensteiner (1987) proposed a two-phase model of the bereavement process as experienced by the parents of children with disabilities. They posited that within the first phase, parents experience an emotional roller-coaster ride by moving circularly in the stages of impact–denial–grief and sadness. In the second phase, parents successfully integrate the child into their life and experience emotional eruptions that are less frequent and less intense. Thus, with time and 'adequate coping', some parents may move into the second phase of chronic sorrow in which the sorrow does not end, yet becomes less intense and has fewer exacerbations and becomes more bearable.

Since the initial research on parents of children with disabilities, a group of American nursing researchers (the Nursing Consortium of Research on Chronic Sorrow) explored the possibility of chronic sorrow in caregivers in other populations – individuals with chronic illness or life-threatening illnesses and their family caregivers and individuals who have experienced the death of a family member (Eakes et al. 1991). These researchers found that chronic sorrow was evident in 86% of individuals with chronic or life-threatening illnesses and present in 83% of family caregivers and 97% in bereaved individuals. These studies then led to the refinement of the concept and added more specificity to the term and published the middle-range theoretical model of chronic sorrow (Eakes et al. 1998) and defined chronic sorrow as '…the periodic recurrence of permanent pervasive sadness or other grief related experiences associated with a significant loss' (p. 179). Critically, this description focuses on the disparity that exists between a person's reality and the idealized, for example, the perfect child, or when a gap exists between the desired relationship and the actual one. Moreover, this sadness and sorrow persists as long as the disparity exists.

A critical attribute of chronic sorrow is that the sadness is not continuous but episodic, triggered by critical times in the child's development. These triggers force the parents to realise the disparity between their own child and the child that they had hoped for. According to Olshansky (1962), it is this constant reminder of the child's differences that prevents the family from gaining a final resolution of their feelings. This disparity often occurs with *trigger events* or milestones such as circumstances, events or situations that bring the disparity into focus or exacerbate the experience of the disparity; see Table 5.2.

Research indicates a fundamental difference between chronic sorrow and clinical depression, emphasising the importance of nurses familiarising themselves with the distinctions between the two and cautioning against labelling the family member as being depressed when individuals are experiencing continuous grief, which can lead to misdiagnosis, mistreatment and poor management of chronic sorrow. Fundamentally, whilst depression can lead to a non-functioning state, chronic sorrow does not interfere with normal everyday functioning. Also, it is important to understand and make distinction between normal grief following death and sadness associated with chronic sorrow. Hogan et al. (2006) argue that chronic sorrow is adaptive grieving and is to be distinguished from complicated grief. This normal grief reaction to the ongoing experience of loss may result from one catastrophic event, such as a debilitating medical diagnosis and trauma or a series or progression of events and symptoms, for example, MS.

Within the United Kingdom, children under the age of 18 years with developmental, behavioural or emotional disabilities are estimated to be around 7% of all children (i.e. 0.9 million) (Department of Work and Pensions 2014). Improvements in technology and medical care have also meant that the lifespan of children with disabilities is advancing, along with

Table 5.2 Trigger events for chronic sorrow

Trigger	Examples
Comparison with norms	Comparison with the norms and the realisation of the disparity between their situation and societal norms Engagement in normal activities, e.g., sports activities Certain jobs out of bounds, e.g., armed forces with physical disability
Milestones	Milestones that cannot be achieved due to the person's condition Childhood milestones such as learning to walk, talk and feed themselves The fitting of a new wheelchair or adaptations in the home Critical periods such as starting a new school Passing of certain birthdays, e.g., 18 or 21 Anniversary of the diagnosis or accident Change in treatment for moving from oral medication to injections
Management of crisis	Situations that challenge the condition or treatment options, such as an exacerbation of the illness requiring hospitalisation or change and/ or need for additional treatment Management crisis and events that invite comparisons with the norms Emotional response that is recurrent and intensifies during initial presentation of illness, developmental transitions, increasing healthcare demands and periods of new or worsened symptoms
Realisation of unending caregiving	Events that bring to mind the realisation of unending caregiving, e.g., hospitalisation or deterioration in the person's condition to the point of dependency Realisation of the anticipated lifestyle and their unending caregiving responsibilities

children who otherwise would have died in the past but are now surviving. For example, children with hydrocephalus, often associated with conditions such as spinal bifida, would have died before ventricular shunting was established in the 1940s, but now it is a relatively minor, routine surgical procedure. Also, advances in technologies such as fetal genetic screening and testing and the increasing pursuit of the 'perfect' baby (Rothwell 2000), may result in some parents who have a disabled child to feel that they are unable to express their sorrow as they may feel disconnected from those with 'normal' children, and feel isolated from their friends, relatives and community.

Despite Olshansky providing an understanding of the concept in relation to parents of disabled children during the past 20 years, a growing number of published studies support the existence of chronic sorrow in parents of children with various identified physical disabilities (Hobdell 2004), significant developmental disabilities (Kearney and Griffin 2001) and mental illness (Mohr and Regan-Kubinski 2001). Chronic sorrow has been documented in a variety of acute and chronic childhood diseases such as diabetes mellitus (Bowes et al. 2008), sickle cell disease (Northington 2000), epilepsy (Hobdell et al. 2007; Wang 2008), neuromuscular disease (Bettle and Latimer 2009), Wilson disease (Ma et al. 2012) and cancer (Nikfarid et al. 2015).

Similarly, chronic sorrow has also been documented in caregivers of adults with chronic and progressive diseases and spouses of persons with AD (Mayer 2001), Parkinson's disease

(Hainsworth et al. 1994; Lindgren 1996), severe chronic diseases (Ahlstrom 2007) and MS (Eakes 1995; Leidstrom et al. 2008). Notably, most of these studies are small in sample size and largely carried out on people with invisible diseases. Other chronic conditions have the potential for family members to experience symptoms of chronic sorrow, for example, where caregivers experience losses and disappointment as a result of their loved ones' lifestyle changes (i.e. limitations and restrictions on activities that they previously were able to do) as a result of the disease process. In summary, previous studies suggest that nurses caring for families in a wide variety of settings need to be aware of high potential for chronic sorrow to occur and therefore cannot ignore this phenomenon.

Assessment of Chronic Sorrow

To avoid mismanagement of chronic sorrow, referral to an appropriate healthcare professional for assessment is important. However, no instrument is available to diagnose chronic sorrow. Failure to recognise chronic sorrow may lead to increased distress in someone who is already experiencing distress. Furthermore, an appreciation of families experiencing chronic sorrow and its potential impact on their ability to care for their family members is critical to family nursing.

Two instruments to measure chronic sorrow have been developed. The first, and the most commonly used, is the Burke/NCRCS Chronic Sorrow Questionnaire, adapted from Burke's (1989) Chronic Sorrow Questionnaire, which uses a set of 16 Likert-style questions rating feelings of disparity, grief, triggers and characteristics of chronic sorrow and aims to determine the impact of loss on the individual. The second is Kendall's chronic sorrow instrument (2005), an 18-item tool using a 7-point Likert scale. These tools not only provide nurses with the opportunity to assess and evaluate the levels of sorrow in family caregivers but also to identify supportive interventions at the appropriate time for those experiencing it. Research suggests that both women and men experience chronic sorrow, although some studies show parental differences (Hobdell 2004). However, each person is distinct in their appreciation of the situations and events; thus, each family member should be assessed separately. In the framework of chronic sorrow identified by Burke and Hainsworth (1998) two antecedents or prerequisites to chronic sorrow have been identified:

1. Single event of a living loss is experienced.
2. Unresolved disparity resulting from the loss.

By being aware of these two antecedents, nurses can identify more readily those families suffering from chronic sorrow. Moreover, nurses need to recognize that caregivers may experience chronic sorrow subsequent to a loss experienced at any point during the lifespan. Chronic sorrow can affect the caregiver's coping ability and can be exacerbated by the pile-up of stressors such as missing key developmental milestones coupled with hospitalisation time. The family's ability to cope with chronic sorrow is dependent on the family's ability to adjust and adapt to their child's illness.

Key Points

- Chronic sorrow is a normal response to an ongoing disparity resulting from a loss.
- Chronic sorrow is experienced cyclically as long as the disparity exists.
- The phenomenon exists in a wide range of family members living with chronic illnesses and diseases.

Impact on Family Roles and Relationships

As caregiving takes place within a relationship, it goes without saying that caregiving will impact the relationship between the carer and care recipient. The carer's motivation and the meaning that they assign to their caregiving role can also have an impact on their relationship and on caregiving outcomes (see Chapter 2). Moreover, this relationship can change over time. Furthermore, as all family members are psychologically and behaviourally connected, it goes without saying that any disruption will affect all family members. It is important to remember that every family system is unique and thus not all families react in the same way, as we have seen in previous chapters.

Family illness or trauma dramatically disrupts the integrity of the family system's equilibrium and the roles performed within the family unit. However, changes may also impact upon the family structure and functioning alongside the changes of concepts of self. These changes in the context of the family stress process are referred to as secondary stressors, or 'spillover effects' as Pearlin et al. (1990) articulate. Consequently, these changes reverberate through the whole family; for example, a wife who customarily provided emotional support to all family members, but following her husband's injury, no longer has the time to provide the same amount of emotional nurturance to other family members who may also suffer. However, other family members may fill the gap; the family reorganises and adapts to manage the shifting needs. Those families that remain in their role or are unable or unwilling to compensate for the decreased functioning of the injured member become unhealthy and dysfunctional. Family relationships may become strained; for example, family members who use all their energy to manage their stress often have little capacity to deal with family relationships. Furthermore, changing family membership creates ambiguity about who is in and who is out of the family, derailing family dynamics, as we have seen in boundary ambiguity discussed previously.

The degree to which individuals may react may be dependent upon the uniqueness of an individual's role and function within the family. In an effort to reduce the negative impact on family functioning, researchers have attempted to identify variables that disrupt family functioning and these include characteristics of the injured, such as neurobehavioral problems, the family and their coping resources. Psychosocial adjustment within the family may also be affected by a range of antecedent variables, i.e., premorbid psychosocial variables, personal and environmental resources and situational factors. Assessment of family function will be explored in more detail in Chapter 7.

Role Changes

Roles within the family quickly change, and may even be permanent, in the event of acute illness or trauma. The impact of sudden role changes within the family can have far-reaching consequences, such as children finding it difficult to adjust to the sudden impact of an ill parent. Some may lose a role, such as wife or partner, but equally, there may be role gain or acquisition when they acquire the role of caregiver. Literature would suggest that partners experience significantly more role changes than parents; this may be because parents' roles are either familiar or exaggerations of existing roles or prior roles. These role changes entail the caregiver to take on a new identity, that of a 'carer' rather than losing their original identity. Thus, the other role identities that a carer may hold, such as wife and mother or husband and father, are not lost but hidden as the carer's role takes precedence. As identity theory postulates, taking on a new identity involves all the cultural and social norms of behaviour associated with the role. However, some caregivers may view their role as an extension of their existing roles rather than as a discrete one. In some circumstances, role reversal may occur as a mother or wife assumes the role of primary breadwinner, when their husband has to give up work due to illness. What is critical to a family caregiver's ability to adjust to these role changes or situational role transitions as they are sometimes referred to is the availability of appropriate and effective support, as we will see in Chapter 6.

What is perhaps unique about caregiving is that as caregivers take on the task of caring, their own identity gets consumed and lost. Several researchers have examined the process of negotiating and reconstructing identity as a person adopts the role of carer. This reconstructing and reorganising in the family is not without stress. As the caregiving activities increase, the person becomes absorbed or engulfed by the caregiving role and a loss of self may be experienced as they live in the shadows of their loved one. Skaff and Pearlin (1992) found that loss of self, defined as a loss of identity that comes about as a result of engulfment in the caregiver role, was common amongst spouses, females and younger caregivers of relatives with AD. According to Aneshensel and colleagues (1992), 'role captivity' refers to situations in which caregivers are unwilling incumbents of their social role as a carer or are entrapped, a role that they did not seek. Literature suggests that stressors that exacerbate this feeling of role captivity include loss of attachment, challenging behaviours of the care recipient and role overload and are alleviated by institutionalisation.

Family changes in relationship dynamics and family functioning are perhaps the most profound in ABI (e.g. stroke and TBI) and degenerative diseases such as dementia and other conditions where their loved ones change significantly and are no longer the 'same person'; i.e., they are caring for a person who is markedly altered from the individual he or she married. These relationship changes and losses experienced between caregiver and care receiver are perhaps amongst the saddest consequences of caregiving. Evidence suggests that in some cases this may result in family dysfunction and relationship failure or marital discord and eventually breakup. The unique challenges faced by families after ABI have been extensively detailed in the research literature with evidence suggesting that spouses of ABI persons who exhibit challenging behaviour have increased marital difficulties, including separation and divorce (Wood and Yurdakul 1997; Katz et al. 2005). The intense and binding nature of the marital relationship makes it particularly unique and vulnerable to negative changes such as a spouse's illness. Caregiving may create intra-role conflict between the caregiver and the marital partner as the couple handles stress in different ways. More specifically, the impact of caregiving on marital relationships can vary. For some, the experience brings them closer together, with open communication and sharing of responsibilities, whilst for others, there is a reallocation of roles, loss of a reciprocal relationship (including financial decision-making), loss of intimacy and a loss of partnership (Braine 2011). This may lead to loneliness, further compounding the negative experience of caregiving.

The dynamic nature of caregiving also makes uncertainty a key feature. Although the term 'uncertainty' may be perceived as being synonymous with ambiguity, Boss (2007) makes it clear that these are not the same constructs. Uncertainty permeates the lives of all family carers and can arise from many sources, including

- Their loved ones' illness or disease trajectory
- The complexity of healthcare
- Inadequate information about their loved ones' condition and treatment
- Role changes and relationships in the family
- Uncertainty about future tasks and responsibilities

The unfamiliarity, unpredictability and inability to make sense of the situation along with the complex nature of caring for a loved one all contribute to a sense of uncertainty. Literature indicates that uncertainty reduces the ability to adjust and adapt. This is key to why reducing uncertainty should be a target for interventions in supporting families and carers. It also affects the carer's sense of hope as uncertainty paralyses hope. Uncertainty is a significant psychological stressor and those who are less tolerant to uncertainty are at greater risk of negative consequences. The sudden nature of some condition and diseases, for example, trauma and acute illness, poses particular challenges. The unbounded, unpredictable and fragile nature of some care recipient's conditions creates uncertainty of the future not just for the carer but also for their loved one. Moreover, family caregivers may feel uncertain about how well they are meeting the needs of other family members.

Key Points

- Caregiving may mean role losses and role gains.
- Caregiving changes role relationship and family functioning.
- A greater awareness is required of the factors that lead to the breakdown of personal relationship when caregiving is involved.

Loss of Couplehood

Whilst the literature in the field of dementia has tended to focus on stress and burden as a consequence of caregiving, a growing interest is emerging that views the caregiver's experience more holistically. This view has led researchers to explore the unique nature of the intimate relationship between a caregiving spouse and his or her partner with dementia as they adapt to the demands of caring whilst experiencing significant losses in their couple relationship. Ade-Ridder and Kaplan (1993, p. 20) describe this relationship 'couplehood' and defined this as 'feelings of belonging to a couple unit'. Kaplan et al. (1995) later explored this sense of belonging in more detail in their study of wives and their perceptions of their relationship with their husbands with dementia who resided in a nursing home and developed a typology of couplehood: (1) no couplehood or 'unmarried marrieds', (2) low couplehood or 'husbandless wives' and (3) high couplehood or 'till death do us part'. These categories of relationships can be best understood in terms of the extent to which the couples have feelings of 'we-ness' rather than 'I-ness'. According to Evans and Lee (2014), couplehood is a broad concept that covers the overall relational experience of separation caused by dementia. Couplehood has also been described as an active process in which couples take part to sustain their couplehood through maintaining affection and reciprocity (Hellstrom and Lund 2007).

Not only has the research in this area focused solely on dementia couples, it is primarily focused on couples living at home. In a systematic review, Evans and Lee (2014) explored the impact of dementia on partner/spouse relationships and reported that the couples' relationships changed, particularly in terms of the nature of their relationship, reciprocity in their partnership and companionship, and that this diminished as the dementia advanced. In a meta-analysis of couples' shared experience of dementia, Wadham et al. (2015) report that the couples strive to maintain their shared sense of couplehood was a key issue. Others have reported similar findings; for example, Førsund et al.'s (2014) Norwegian-grounded theory revealed that spouses lost their sense of couplehood and felt alone when their dementia partner was living under institutional care. The effect on marital relationships as a result of one partner leaving home and moving to a residential/nursing home facility has been labelled 'married widowhood' by Rollins et al. (1985), which epitomises this sense of loss of couplehood. Adjustment to the institutionalisation of their partner and loss of identity as a functioning couple creates a unique grieving process, as we have discussed earlier in terms of ambiguous loss and anticipatory grief.

Couplehood has not been researched within other chronic illnesses and conditions, but it has been based on the concept that carers of people with cognitive impairment from other disease processes such as ABI (e.g. TBI and stroke), degenerative diseases such as Parkinson's disease, MS and mental illness may be given important consideration. Changes in the cognitive abilities of a person with dementia or acquired brain injury (e.g. TBI) mean changes in roles and responsibilities, which often result in an imbalance in the relationship, creating a reduced togetherness and a sense of becoming 'I' rather than 'we'.

The uniqueness of the spouse relationship highlights the importance of acknowledging the vulnerability and uniqueness of their situations when one member becomes ill and there is a need for nurses to understand this delicate relationship. The severity of some spouses' experiences, of losing their sense of couplehood, emphasises the need for nurses to understand the relational effects of illness so that a more holistic approach to care for both members of the dyad can be provided. Awareness of how these experiences could fluctuate and be situational is also important, and Kaplan's typology provides a useful means of understanding the different experiences of spouses. Again, this highlights that not all spousal carers should be viewed alike as a homogenous group. By listening carefully to how a spouse talks about their partner, nurses can gain an insight into how they perceive couplehood and therefore their specific needs. For example, a spousal carer may resist labelling themselves a 'carer' but rather view the changes in their role and relationship as part of their ongoing relationship with their partner, indicating their shared sense of couplehood.

Identifying services in which the couple can be together acknowledging and accommodating this concept of couplehood should be considered by nurses, particularly those working in the community. By working proactively with couples, nurses may be able to enhance their strategies for sustaining couplehood and maintaining involvement. Equally important is the identification of those couples that are not close and thus may require additional support and/or be provided with information so that they can explore alternative caring arrangements, such as institutional care. Crucially, in this situation the spouse may only want to play the role of visitor, and so unrealistic demands to participate in care for such spouses should be avoided. As nurses, we should not judge relationships per se but be aware of differences and opportunities for offering support.

Positive Outcomes of Caregiving

Every caregiver who faces adversity will react differently – some will react with manifestation of stress, as we have already discussed, whereas others will show resilience and thrive. Although there continues to be keen interest on the negative impact on health morbidity, increased attention has been given to the fact that not all caregivers experience negative health outcomes. There is mounting evidence that caregivers identify long-term positive benefits from the complexities and dilemmas posed by caregiving. Indeed, they are not all overly burdened with their multiple role expectations, and caregiving may be a catalyst for reprioritisation and positive life change. In Chapter 1, we highlighted different types of carers, and in some instances, e.g., compound carers, carers are thought to reach a threshold that enables them to cope with and manage their role. It is also plausible that positive consequences, such as positive growth, reward and satisfaction, gratification, increased sense of mastery, a sense of giving something back and higher levels of subjective well-being, may buffer the negative effects of caregiving. Moreover, both negative and positive consequences of providing care may exist simultaneously. However, nurses need to be mindful that not all caregivers can find benefit and growth from their experiences, and if they do, this does not mean that they are not experiencing distress and suffering as well. The following paragraphs will explore some of these positive aspects of caregiving in more detail.

These positive aspects of coping can be attributed to the Lazurus and Folkman's stress and coping paradigm and the revised Folkman's transactional model of stress (1997) which emphasise the positive emotions that can arise from stressors even when there is no resolution for the event. The model emphasises the importance of an individual's appraisal of stressors and the extent to which they present a threat or benefit. In Folkman's model, the individual's perception of the stressor is important along with the ongoing appraisal of what the stressor means to that individual and whether they have necessary resources to cope with it. For example, when faced with a spouse suffering a sudden debilitating ABI, e.g. stroke, the individual assesses the significance of the event which may be perceived as stressful, positive and beneficial, or challenging or irrelevant. The carer, through cognitive processing, reframes the negative experience into new patterns of self and their future. Whether a family caregiver experiences caregiving as positive or satisfying can be influenced by a number of factors, including caregiver characteristics, such as having a positive outlook on their caregiving challenges perceiving them to be less stressful than those with a negative outlook, and the unique caregiving situation.

Although the phenomenon of positive growth that can be found in suffering is not new, systematic investigation especially within the field of clinical health psychology is an emerging area of empirical study. Over the past 20 years, researchers have also shifted their focus from the negative to the positive effects of family caregiving, albeit this being a relatively slim body of research. This focus provides a more balanced view of caregiving and can help nurses to understand the complexities of caring and aid in the development of more appropriate interventions to support family caregivers. Furthermore, assessments of caregiver needs should include positive and negative aspects of caregiving. These assessments may help nurses to identify what caregiver's value along with services and support that they might find helpful so that this can be enhanced.

Within the literature, several terms have been associated with the positive attributes derived from caregiving. Hunt (2003) identified and defined five different positive conceptualizations of the construct of caregiving in order to provide greater clarity: (1) caregiver esteem or confidence as a direct result of caregiving; (2) up-lifts of caregiving [daily] events that make one feel good, joyful, or glad, or satisfied; (3) caregiver satisfaction, (4) finding or making meaning, i.e. assessing positive aspects of and ways to find [higher levels of] meaning through caregiving; and (5) gain in the caregiving experience or positive return from the caregiving experience (pp. 29–30).

Researchers have also used a variety of constructs and theories to explain the perceived positive and meaningful consequences of trauma or severe adversity in an individual's life, including stress-related growth (Park 1996), PTG (Tedeschi and Calhoun 1996) and adversarial growth (Linley and Joseph 2004). Although these terms are used interchangeably within the literature, we offer a brief overview of these terms.

Tedeschi and Colhoun (1996, 2004) coined the construct *post-traumatic growth* to describe positive psychological changes as a result of highly challenging life circumstances.

A key component of PTG is that exposure to trauma or similar event needs to accompany or be followed by a perceived threat to the individual's well-being. However, it is not the major life crisis itself that is responsible for the growth, but the cognitive processing after the crisis that brings about the growth. At the core of PTG is the notion that the assumptions people hold about life and the world become shattered by a severe adversity or unintentional change, which is called a *seismic event*. This disrupts cognitive schematic structures (units of one's understanding of oneself and the world) which once provided meaning, understanding and decision-making capacity (Tedeschi and Calhoun 2004). This is followed by a period of reorganisation where the potential for growth occurs by the change mechanism of rumination (turning things over in the mind or recurrent thinking), which initiates the growth process. Thus, PTG is based on models of human change and is both an active process and an outcome. At this point, it is important to note that PTG acts like a springboard in that the individual is propelled into growth and development which goes beyond managing and coping with adversity. In this regard, PTG is unlike resilience in which an individual copes well with adversity but does not undergo transformation. In other words, they thrive.

Over the last two decades, research has indicated that these positive changes occur in five main areas: new possibilities, relationships with others, individuals' perception of self, philosophy of life and spiritual change. PTG is often measured with the PTG inventory (Tedeschi and Calhoun 1996) devised to assess these positive changes; it provides a total score from 21 items and 5 sub-scores based on the five areas of change and has demonstrated good validity in several studies.

Initially, PTG was studied in survivors of traumatic experiences of war or natural disasters, but since then there has been an increased interest in positive growth in caregivers, in particular adult caregivers, although this is limited. Linley and Joseph (2004) documented in a review of positive change following trauma and adversity that positive change can result from a wide range of situations including caregivers of cancer patients and parenting a child with disabilities. Most studies use the term PTG, and despite the early PTG model arguing that a seismic event needs to occur, illness and disease can also threaten to dramatically change the lives of families and caregivers. PTG has been reported in adult caregivers of people with physical health illness (Mock and Boener 2010), parenting children with autism (Phelps et al. 2009), cancer (Thormbre et al. 2010; Cormio et al. 2014), stroke (Haley et al. 2009), AD (Sanders 2005; Peacock et al. 2010; Cheng et al. 2015) and mental illness (Chen and Greenberg 2004; Sanders and Szymanski 2013). Mackenzie and Greenwood's (2012) systematic review of stroke caregivers' positive experiences confirmed not only the existence of positive experiences of the long-term illness but also an increase in self-esteem and feelings of being appreciated. In an earlier exploration of 560 caregivers of patients with schizophrenia, Chen and Greenberg (2004) found positive gains to be prevalent with 70% of the caregivers being more sensitive towards the person with disabilities and more than 50% reporting a greater sense of inner strength and greater intimacy with other family members. The researchers also identified the importance of support in facilitating personal growth and enhancing interpersonal relationships.

Two meta-analyses and a systematic review of PTG studies revealed certain variables associated with PTG that provide some valuable insights for supporting families and caregivers. First, Prati and Pietrantoni's (2009) meta-analysis of 103 studies of PTG concluded that optimism, social support, spirituality, acceptance coping, reappraisal coping, religious coping and seeking support coping were associated with PTG amongst adults. Second, Vishnevsky et al.'s (2010) meta-analysis of 70 studies that examined gender differences in PTG concluded that women reported more PTG than men and that PTG scores amongst women increased with age. Meyerson et al.'s (2011) systematic review of 22 studies of PTG in children and adolescents not only reported growth experiences as a result of trauma but also similar influencing variables such as social support and religious support.

Further research with younger populations including young carers is necessary to determine the nature of positive growth and the influencing factors. In a recent systematic review of PTG in parents and paediatric patients with serious illness by Picoraro et al. (2014) not only found evidence of PTG in parents of medical trauma but concluded that this understudied and inadequately understood phenomena requires further research. Given that the literature to date has in the main focused on patients, further studies are required to explore the possible influences of specific illness on positive aspects of caregiving along with caregiver factors such as relationship with the care recipient, age, gender, culture and ethnicity. This will help healthcare professionals identify what factors mediate the presence of positive growth in caregivers and what interventions may promote it.

Two main personal characteristics have been associated with the likelihood that a person can make positive changes; these include openness to new possibilities and experiences and having an extraversion personality (Linley and Joseph 2004; Tedeschi and Calboun 2004). In addition, the availability of mutually supportive others has been identified as important in aiding PTG. In the PTG model, emotional support (comfort) is thought to aid in contemplating the changes or constructive rumination brought about by the crisis, and the more a person contemplates the change, the more likely they are to grow. In the context of supporting families and caregivers, the use of carer support groups, during which sharing and being with others in similar circumstances happen, may facilitate the ruminative process and thus a willingness to see new perspectives and undergo positive change. For carers who do not report a supportive social network, local support groups may provide an alternative safe social environment that may facilitate constructive rumination. Tedeschi and Calhoun (2004) suggest that this association may be attributed to role that support groups play in generating coping skills and adaptability. Thus, social support acts as a buffer.

Synonymous with PTG is the term *adversarial growth* coined by the psychologists Linley and Joseph (2004) to cover all aspects of positive changes that occur following adversity. Linley and Joseph (2004) suggest that growth can also take place through more gradual breakdown and rebuilding of the assumptive world. Like PTG, the researchers argue that adversarial growth is a process and is influenced by the subjective experience of the event rather than the event itself. The construct stress-related growth (Park 1996), however, includes events that are not perceived as being threatening as in PTG. Other terms are evident in the literature such as positive adaption, thriving and perceived benefits. What seems to be common in all these constructs and theories is that positive growth results from the struggle with a stressful situation or adversity, and stress seems necessary for the positive growth to occur.

Intervention to support families and carers can focus on the positive benefits of caregiving along with an emphasis on social support and other mechanism to reduce the negative effects or caregiving. On an individual basis, focus on both the strengths and weaknesses of a carer are important for interventions. Nurses who only view caregiving as negative limit their abilities to help and support positive factors and thus improve their caregiving experience.

Key Points

- Caregivers can experience growth and personal development as a result of their caregiving role.
- Nurses need to take into account both positive and negative effects of caregiving to enable a more holistic view of the caregiver's experience.
- Assessment for adaptation to the caregiving experience should incorporate both positive and negative indices of adjustment.
- Further research is needed to explore the possible social and cultural factors that can harness and facilitate positive growth in families and caregivers.

Chapter Summary

Caregiving can be burdensome, demanding and unpredictable and can place caregivers at risk for deleterious effect on their health and well-being, including physically, emotionally and psychologically. This chapter has attempted to provide an overview of some of the many consequences of caregiving, which often go unrecognised as the main focus tends to be on the care recipients. Both the negative and positive effects of caregiving on both the individual and family as a whole have been discussed. Burden, social isolation and loss are some of the main negative consequences of caregiving. Loss and grief are constant insidious companions for caregivers. Not only is this saddening, but it is also a reminder to all of us that it is often unnoticed, unrecognised and non-finite in nature and thus should be an important consideration in supporting families and carers. The literature continues to evolve in this area, but what is striking is that family caregivers' loss is profound and multidimensional. Several factors have been explored that link psychological health and well-being of caregivers, including carer's demographics, the caregiving process and contextual factors.

We have found that the published literature on the positive effects of caregiving is relatively limited; nonetheless, it offers some balance to the all too often view that caregiving is a negative experience. Given that we are facing an ageing population and huge technological advances in medicine and healthcare, the likelihood of caring for survivors of severe trauma and illness will increase. Therefore, understanding both these aspects of caregiving will become increasingly important to us all. Nurses need to focus not just on protecting carer's health and well-being, because their caregiving demands place them at high risk of adverse effects, but also in helping carers to learn how to be competent and safe informal carers so as to protect their loved ones from unnecessary harm.

Throughout this chapter, a range of screening and assessment tools have been illuminated, although predominantly used in research and psychology, to assess specific elements/features associated with the impact of being a caregiver. Whilst some of these may not be used by nurses, we feel it is important that nurses have some awareness and knowledge of the various tools. For some nurses, such tools may be important adjuncts to their practice depending upon the role of the nurse and the setting within which they work. Moreover, if nurses recognise psychological, behavioural and physiological effects of caregiving, there may be more opportunities for preventative health.

Much of the research on the impact of injury and/or illness on the family and individual have focused on a 'snapshot' of a certain point in time. However, the impact of caregiving on the family can be long-lasting and life changing and can change with time. Further research is needed if we are to understand the full impact of caregiving on all family members, especially over time. A clearer understanding of the factors that influence psychological and physiological responses to environmental stressors such as caregiving is also warranted. Men, whether husbands or sons, are notably underrepresented in family caregiving, yet they play an important role in caregiving. Exploring gender difference across diverse caregiver populations in more detail may provide a more balanced view of the impact of caregiving.

Healthcare systems, policymakers and healthcare professionals such as nurses need to recognise the importance of maintaining the health and well-being of carers in light of the vital role that they play in healthcare. As nurses spend a great deal of time with patients and their families, they are in a unique position to address these issues through support and appropriate intervention; see Chapter 6.

References

Adelman RD, Tmanova LL, Delgado D, Dion S and Lachs MS. (2014) Caregiver burden: A clinical review. *Journal of the American Medical Association* 311(10): 1052–1060.

Ade-Ridder L and Kaplan L. (1993) Marriage spousal caregiving and a husbands move to a nursing home: A changing role for the wife? *Journal of Gerontological Nursing* 19: 13–23.

Ahlstrom G. (2007) Experiences of loss and chronic sorrow in persons with severe chronic illness. *Journal of Clinical Nursing* 16(3A): 76–83.

Al-Gamal E and Long T. (2013) The MM-CGI cerebral palsy: Modification and pretesting of an instrument to measure anticipatory grief in parent who child has cerebral palsy. *Journal of Clinical Nursing* 23: 1810–1819.

Al-Gamal E, Long T and Livesley J. (2009) Development of a modified instrument to measure anticipatory grief in Jordanian parents of children diagnosed with cancer. *Cancer Nursing* 32(3): 211–219.

Aneshensel CS, Pearlin LI and Schuler RH. (1993) Role captivity, and the cessation of caregiving. *Journal of Health and Social Behaviour* 34(1): 54–70.

Archbold PG, Stewart BJ, Greenlick MR and Harvath TA. (1990) Mutually and prepared as predictor of caregiver role strain. *Research in Nursing & Health* 13: 375–384.

Beltrão MRLR, Vasconcelos MGL, Ponte CM and Albuquerque MC. (2007) Childhood cancer: Maternal perceptions and strategies for coping with diagnosis. *Jornal de Pediatria* 83(6): 562–566.

Berkman LF, Glass T, Brissette I and Seeman TE. (2000) From social integration to health: Durkheim in the new millennium. *Social Science and Medicine* 51: 843–857.

Bettle A and Latimer M. (2009) Maternal coping and adaptation: A case study examination of chronic sorrow in caring for an adolescent with a progressive neuromuscular disease. *Canadian Journal of Neuroscience Nursing* 31(4): 15–21.

Biddle B. (1986) Recent developments in role theory. *Annual Review of Sociology* 12: 67–92.

Blackburn CM, Spencer CM and Read JM. (2010) Prevalence of childhood disability and the characteristics and circumstances of disabled children in the UK: Secondary analysis of the Family Resources Survey. *BMC Pediatrics* 10: 21.

Blandin K and Peplin R. (2015) Dementia grief: A theoretical model of a unique grief experience. *Dementia* 1–12, [online] 15 April 2015. doi: 10.1177/1471301215581081.

Blieszner R, Roberto KA, Wilcox KL, Barham EJ and Winston BL. (2007) Dimensions of ambiguous loss in couples coping with mild cognitive impairment. *Family Relations* 56(2): 196–209.

Boss P. (1977) A clarification of the concepts of psychological father presence in families experiencing ambiguity of boundary. *Journal of Marriage and Family* 39: 141–151.

Boss P. (1987) Family stress. In: M. B. Sussman and S. K. Steinmetz (Eds.) *Handbook of Marriage and Family.* New York: Plenum, pp. 695–723.

Boss P. (1999) *Ambiguous Loss.* Cambridge, MA: Harvard University Press.

Boss P. (2002) *Family Stress Management: A Contextual Approach*, 2nd ed. Thousand Oaks, CA: Sage Publications Inc.

Boss P. (2004) Ambiguous loss research, theory, and practice: Reflections after 9/11. *Journal of Marriage and Family* 66(3): 551–566.

Boss P. (2006) *Loss Trauma and Resilience.* New York: W.W. Norton & Company.

Boss P. (2007) Ambiguous loss theory: Challenges for scholars and practitioners. *Family Relations* 56: 105–111.

Boss P. (2010) The trauma and complicated grief of ambiguous loss. *Pastoral Psychology* 59(2): 137–145.

Boss P and Couden BA. (2002) Ambiguous loss from chronic physical illness: Clinical interventions with individuals, couples, and families. *Journal of Clinical Psychology* 58(11): 1351–1360.

Boss P and Greenberg J. (1984) Family boundary ambiguity: A new variable in family stress theory. *Family Process* 23: 535–546.

Boss P and Yeats J. (2014) Ambiguous loss: A complicated type of grief when loved ones disappear. *Bereavement Care* 33(2): 63–69.

Bowes S, Lowes L, Warner J and Gregory JW. (2008) Chronic sorrow in parents of children with type 1 diabetes. *Journal of Advanced Nursing* 65(5): 992–1000.

Braine ME. (2010) Acquired brain injury and the emotional, behavioural and cognitive sequelae: The family experience, Unpublished thesis. Salford, UK: University of Salford.

Braine ME. (2011) The experience of living with a family member with challenging behaviour post acquired brain injury. *Journal of Neuroscience Nursing* 43(3): 156–164.

Bruce EJ and Schultz CL. (2001) *Nonfinite Loss and Grief.* Sydney, New South Wales, Australia: Paul H. Brooke Publishing Co.

Burke ML, Eakes GG and Hainsworth MA. (1989) Milestones of chronic sorrow: Perspectives of chronically.

Burke ML. (1989) Chronic sorrow in mothers of school-age children with a myelomeningocele disability. Doctoral dissertation, Boston University, Boston, MA.

Burton L, Newsom J, Schulz R, Hirsch CH and German PS. (1997) Preventive health behaviors among spousal caregivers. *Preventative Medicine* 26(2): 162–169.

Cacioppo JT, Cacioppo S and Boomsma DI. (2014) Evolutionary mechanisms for loneliness. *Cognition and Emotion* 28: 3–21.

Cacioppo JT, Cacioppo S, Cacioppo JP and Cole SW. (2015) The neuroendocrinology of social isolation. *Annual Review of Psychology* 66: 9.1–9.35.

Carrà G, Cazzullo CL and Clerici M. (2012) The association between expressed emotion, illness severity and subjective burden of care in relatives of patients with schizophrenia. Findings from an Italian population. *BMC Psychiatry* 12: 140.

Carter JH, Lyons KS, Lindauer A and Malcom J. (2012) Pre-death grief in Parkinson's caregivers: A pilot survey-based study. *Parkinsonism and Related Disorders* 18(Suppl. 3): S15–S18.

Caspi A, Harringto HL, Moffitt TE, Milnes BJ and Poulton R. (2007) Socially isolated children 20 years later: Risk of cardiovascular disease. *Archives of Pediatrics & Adolescent Medicine* 160(8): 805–811.

Chan D, Livingston G, Jones L and Sampson EL. (2013) Grief reactions in dementia carers: A systematic review. *International Journal of Geriatric Psychiatry* 28(1): 1–17.

Chen F and Greenberg JS. (2004) A positive aspect of caregiving: The influence of social support on caregivers gains for family members of relatives with Schizophrenia. *Community Mental Health Journal* 40(5): 423–435.

Cheng S, Mak APM, Lau RWL, Ng NSS and Man LCM. (21 January 2015) Voices of Alzheimer caregivers on positive aspects of caregiving. *The Gerontologist*. pii: gnu118.

Chiambretto P, Moroni L, Guarnerio C, Bertolotti G and Prigerson HG. (2010) Prolonged grief and depression in caregivers of patients in vegetative state. *Brain Injury* 24: 581–588.

Clark MS, Bond MJ and Hecker JR. (2007) Environmental stress, psychological stress and allostatic load. *Psychology, Health & Medicine* 12(1): 18–30.

Clausen JA and Yarrow MR. (1955) The impact of mental illness on the family. *Journal of Socials Issues* 11: 3–64.

Cormio C, Romito F, Viscanti G, Turaccio M, Lorusso V and Mattioli V. (2012) Psychological well-being and posttraumatic growth in caregivers of cancer patients. *Frontiers in Psychology* 4(5): 1342.

Corr CA, Nabe CM and Corr DM. (1997) *Death and Dying, Life and Living.* 2nd edition. Pacific Grove, CA: Brooks/Cole Publishing Company.

Conde-Sala JL, Garre-Olmo J, Turro-Garriga O, Vilalta-Franch J and Lopez-Pousa S. (2010) Differential features of burden between spouse and adult-child caregivers of patients with Alzheimer's disease: An exploratory comparative design. *International Journal of Nursing Studies* 47(10): 1262–1273.

Copley MF and Bodensteiner JB. (1987) Chronic sorrow in families of disabled children. *Journal of Child Neurology* 2: 67–70.

Damrosch SP and Perry LA. (1989) Chronic sorrow in children with Down's syndrome. *Nursing Research* 38: 25–30.

D'Antonio J. (2014) Caregiver grief and anticipatory mourning. *Journal of Hospice & Palliative Nursing* 16: 99–104.

Del-Pino-Casado R, Cold-Osuna A, Moral Palomino PA and Pancorbo-Hidalgo PL. (2011) Coping and subjective burden in caregivers of older relatives: A quantitative systematic review. *Journal of Advanced Nursing* 67(11): 2311–2322.

Denno MS, Gillard PJ, Graham GD, DiBonaventura M, Goren A, Varon SF and Zorowitz R. (2013) Anxiety and depression associated with caregiver burden in caregivers of stroke survivors with spasticity. *Archives of Physical Medicine and Rehabilitation* 94(9): 1731–1736.

Department of Health. (2012) *Caring for Our Future: Reforming Care and Support.* London, UK: The Stationary Office Limited.

Department of Work and Pensions. (2014) *Family Resources Survey United Kingdom 2012–13.* London, UK: Department of Work and Pensions HM UK.

Diwan S, Hougham GW and Sachs GA. (2009) Chronological patterns and issues precipitating grieving over the course of caregiving among family caregivers of persons with dementia. *Clinical Gerontology* 32(4): 358–370.

Doka K. (1989) *Disenfranchised Grief Recognising Hidden Sorrow.* Lexington, MA: Lexington Books.

Doka K. (2002) *Disenfranchised Grief New Directions and Challenges and Strategies for Practice.* Champaign, IL: Research Press.

Drentea P, Clay OJ, Roth DL and Mittelman MS. (2006) Predictors of improvement in social support: Five year effects of a structured intervention for caregivers of spouses with Alzheimer's disease. *Social Science & Medicine* 63(4): 957–967.

Dupuis SL. (2002) Understanding ambiguous loss in the context of dementia care: Adult children's perspectives. *Journal of Gerontological Social Work* 37(2): 93–115.

Eakes GG, Hainsworth ME, Lindgren CL and Burke ML. (1991). Establishing a long-distance research consortium. *Nursing Connections* 4: 51–57.

Eakes GG. (1995) Chronic sorrow in spouses caregivers of individuals with multiple sclerosis. *Journal of Gerontological Nursing* 21(7): 29–33.

Eakes GG, Burke ML and Hainsworth MA. (1998) Middle range theory of chronic sorrow. *Image: Journal of Nursing Scholarship* 30(2): 179–184.

Ennis N, Rosenbloom BN, Canzian S and Toplocvec-Vranic J. (2013) Depression and anxiety in parent versus spouse caregivers of adult patients with traumatic brain injury: A systematic review. *Neuropsychological Rehabilitation* 23(1): 1–18.

Evans D and Lee E. (2014) Impact of dementia on marriage: A qualitative systematic review. *Dementia* 13: 330–349.

Førsund LH, Skovdahl K, Kiik R and Ytrehu SW. (2014) The loss of a shared lifetime: A qualitative study exploring spouses' experiences of losing couplehood with their partner with dementia living in institutional care. *Journal of Clinical Nursing* 24: 121–130.

Fowler NR, Hansen AS, Barnato AE and Garand L. (2013) Association between anticipatory grief and problem solving among family caregivers of persons with cognitive impairment. *Journal of Aging and Health* 25(3): 493–509.

Fraley AM. (1986) Chronic sorrow in parents of premature children. *Children's Health Care* 15: 114–118.

Garard L, Linger JH, Deardorf KE, DeKosky T, Schulz R, Reynolds CF and Dew MA. (2012) Anticipatory grief in new family caregivers of persons with mild cognitive impairment and dementia. *Alzheimer Disease Associated Disorders* 26(2): 159–165.

Garwick AW, Detzner D and Boss P. (1994) Family perceptions of living with Alzheimer's disease. *Family Process* 33(3): 327–340.

Giovannetti AM, Cemiauskaite M, Leonardi DS and Covelli V. (2014) Information caregivers of patients with disorders of consciousness: Experience of ambiguous loss. *Brain Injury* 29(4): 473–480.

Golash T and Powell K. (2003) Ambiguous loss: Managing the dialects of grief associated with premature birth. *Journal of Social and Personal Relationships* 20: 309–334.

Goode W. (1960) Theory of role strain. *American Sociological Review* 25: 483–496.

Grad J and Sainsbury P. (1963) Mental illness and family. *Lancet* 281(7280): 544–547.

Grimby A, Johanson AK and Johansson U. (2015) Anticipatory grief among close relatives of patients with ALS and MS. *Psychology and Behavioral Sciences* 4(3): 125–131.

Haley W, Allen J, Grant J, Clay O, Perkins M and Roth D. (2009) Problems and benefits reported by stroke family caregivers: Results from a prospective epidemiological study. *Stroke* 30: 2129–2133.

Hardy KV and Laszloffy TA. (2005) *Teens Who Hurt: Clinical Interventions to Break the Cycle of Adolescent Violence.* New York: Guilford Press.

Hastrup LH, Van Den Berg B and Gyrd-Hansen D. (2011) Do informal caregivers in mental illness feel more burdened: A comparative study of mental versus somatic illnesses. *Scandinavian Journal of Public Health* 39(6): 598–607.

Hellstrom I and Lund U. (2007) Sustaining "couplehood": Spouses' strategies for living positively with dementia. *Dementia* 6: 383–409.

Hellström I, Nolan M and Lundh U. (2007) Sustaining couplehood: Spouses' strategies for living positively with dementia. *Dementia: International Journal of Social Research and Practice* 6(3): 383–409.

Hill DL. (2006) Sense of belonging as connectedness, American Indian worldview and mental health. *Archives of Psychiatric Nursing* 20(5): 210–216.

Hobdell EF. (2004) Chronic sorrow and depression in parents of children with neural tube defects. *Journal of Neuroscience Nursing* 26(2): 82–94.

Hobdell EF, Grant ML, Valencia I, Mare J, Kothare SV, Legido A and Khurana DS. (2007) Chronic sorrow and coping in families of children with epilepsy. *Journal of Neuroscience Nursing* 39(2): 76–82.

Hoenig J and Hamilton MW. (1966) The schizophrenic patient in the community and the effect on the household. *International Journal of Social Psychiatry* 12: 165–176.

Hogan NS, Worden JW and Schmidt LA. (2006) Considerations in conceptualising complicated grief. *Omega* 529(1): 81–85.

Holley CK and Mast BT. (2009) The impact of anticipatory grief on caregiver burden in dementia caregivers. *The Gerontologist* 49(3): 388–396.

Holt-Lunstad J, Smith TB, Baker M, Harris T and Stephenson D. (2015) Loneliness and social isolation as risk factors for mortality. A meta-analytic review. *Perspectives on Psychological Science* 10: 227–237.

Hunt CK. (2003) Concepts in caregiver research. *Journal of Nursing Scholarship* 35(1): 27–32.

Janevic MR and Connell CM. (2001) Racial, ethnic, and cultural differences in the dementia caregiving experience: Recent findings. *The Gerontologist* 41: 334–347.

Johansson AK and Grimby A. (2012) Anticipatory grief among close relatives of patients at hospice and palliative wards. *American Journal of Hospital & Palliative Medicine* 29(2): 134–138.

Johansson AK and Johannsson U. (2015) Anticipatory grief among close relatives of patients with ALS and MS. *Psychology and Behavioural Sciences* 4(3): 125–131.

Johansson UE and Grimby A. (2014) Anticipatory grief among close relatives of patients with Parkinson disease. *Psychology and Behavioural Sciences* 3(5): 179–184.

Jones PS and Martinson IM. (1992) The experience of bereavement in caregivers of family members with Alzheimer's disease. *IMAGE: Journal of Nursing Scholarship* 24: 172–176.

Kaplan L. (2001) A couplehood typology for spouses of institutionalized persons with Alzheimer's disease: Perceptions of "we"–"I". *Family Relations* 50: 87–98.

Kaplan L, Ade-Ridder L, Hennon CB, Brubaker E and Brubaker T. (1995) Preliminary typology of couplehood for community dwelling wives: 'I' versus 'we'. *International Journal of Aging and Human Development* 40: 317–337.

Katz S, Kravetz S and Grynbaum F. (2005) Wives' coping flexibility, time since husbands' injury and the perceived burden of wives of men with traumatic brain injury. *Brain Injury* 19(1): 59–66.

Kean S. (2010) The experience of ambiguous loss in families of brain injured ICU patients. *Nursing in Critical Care* 15(23): 66–75.

Kearney PM and Griffin T. (2001) Between joy and sorrow: Being a parent of a child with a development disability. *Journal of Advanced Nursing* 34: 582–592.

Kendall LJ. (2005) The experience of living with ongoing loss: Testing the Kendall chronic sorrow instrument. Richmond, VA: Virginia Commonwealth University.

Kim H, Chang M, Rose K and Kim S. (2012) Predictors of caregiver burden in caregivers of individuals with dementia. *Journal of Advanced Nursing* 68(4): 846–855.

Landau J and Hissett J. (2008) Mild traumatic brain injury: Impact on identify and ambiguous loss in the family. *Families, Systems, & Health* 26(1): 69–85.

Lee S, Colditz GA, Berkman LF and Kawachi I. (2003) Caregiving and risk of coronary heart disease in U.S. women: A prospective study. *American Journal of Preventative Medicine* 24(2): 113–119.

Leidstrom E, Isaksson A and Ahlstrom G. (2008) Chronic sorrow in next of kin of patients with Multiple sclerosis. *Journal of Neuroscience Nursing* 40(5): 305–311.

Leonardi M, Giovannetti AM, Pagani M, Raggi A and Sattin D. (2012) Burden and needs of 487 caregivers of patients in vegetative state and in minimally conscious state: Results from a national study. *Brain Injury* 26(10): 1201–1210.

Lezak MD. (1978) Living with the characterologically altered brain injured patient. *Journal of Clinical Psychiatry* 39(7): 592–598.

Lindauer A and Harvath T. (2014) Pre-death grief in the context of dementia caregivers: A concept analysis. *Journal of Advanced Nursing* 70(10): 2196–2207.

Lindemann E. (1944) Symptomatology and the management of acute grief. *American Journal of Psychiatry* 101: 141–148.

Lindgren CL. (1996) Chronic sorrow in persons with Parkinson's disease and their spouses. *Scholarly Inquiry for Nursing Practice* 10(4): 351–366.

Linley PA and Joseph S. (2004) Positive change following trauma and adversity: A review. *Journal of Traumatic Stress* 17: 11–21.

Lubben J, Blozik E, Gillmann G, Iliffe S, von Renteln Kruse W, Beck JC and Stuck AE. (2006) Performance of an abbreviated version of the Lubben Social Network Scale among three European community-dwelling older adult populations. *The Gerontologist* 46(4): 503.

Ma M, Ji Y, Liu Y and Zhang B. (2012) Investigation and intervention on the psychological status of families with Hepatolenticular Degeneration children. *Life Science Journal* 9(2): 910–913.

Mackenzie A and Greenwood N. (2012) Positive experiences of caregiving in stroke: A systematic review. *Disability and Rehabilitation* 34(17): 1413–1422.

Magliano L, McDaid D, Kirkwood S and Berzins K. (2007) Carers and families of people with mental health problems. In: M. Knapp, D. McDaid, E. Mossialos and G. Thornicroft (Eds.) *Mental Health Policy and Practice across Europe*. Berkshire, UK: McGraw-Hill, pp. 374–396.

Marwit SJ, Chibnall JT, Dougherty R, Jenkins C and Shawgo J. (2008) Assessing pre-death grief in cancer caregivers using the Marwit-Meuser Caregiver Grief Inventory (MM-CGI). *Psycho-Oncology* 17(3): 300–303.

Marwit SJ and Kaye PN. (2006) Measuring grief in caregivers of persons with acquired brain injury. *Brain Injury* 20(12–13): 1419–1429.

Marwit SJ and Meuser TM. (2002) Development and initial validation of an inventory to assess grief in caregivers of people with Alzheimer's disease. *The Gerontologist* 42(6): 751–765.

Marwit SJ and Meuser TM. (2005) Development of a short form inventory to assess grief in caregivers of dementia patients. *Death Studies* 29: 191–205.

Mathers CD and Loncar D. (2007) *Neurological Disorders: Public Health Challenges*. Geneva, Switzerland: World Health Organization.

Mayer M. (2001) Chronic sorrow in caregiving spouses of patients with Alzheimer's disease. *Journal of Aging and Identity* 6(1): 49–60.

McKeown L, Porter-Armstrong A and Baxter G. (2004) Caregivers of people with multiple sclerosis: Experiences of support. *Multiple Sclerosis* 10: 219–230.

Meuser TM, Marwit SJ and Sanders S. (2004) Assessing grief in family caregivers. In: K. Doka (Ed.) *Living with Grief: Alzheimer's Disease*. Washington, DC: Hospice Foundation of America, pp. 170–195.

Meyerson DA, Grant KE, Carter J, Smith K and Ryan P. (2011) Posttraumatic growth among children and adolescents: A systematic review. *Clinical Psychology Review* 31(6): 949–964.

Miller B and Cafasso L. (1992) Gender differences in caregiving: Fact or artefact? *The Gerontologist* 32: 598–607.

Mock S and Boener M. (2010) Sense making and benefit finding among patients with amyotrophic lateral sclerosis and their primary caregivers. *Journal of Health Psychology* 15(1): 115–121.

Mohamed S, Rosenheck R, Lyketsos K and Schneider LN. (2010) Caregiver burden in Alzheimer's disease: Cross sectional and longitudinal patient correlates. *American Journal of Geriatric Psychiatry* 18(10): 917–927.

Mohr WK and Regan-Kubinski MJ. (2001) Living in the fallout: Parents' experiences when their child becomes mentally ill. *Archives of Psychiatric Nursing* XV(2): 69–77.

Monin JK and Schulz R. (2010) The effects of suffering in chronically ill older adults on the health and well-being of family members involved in their care. *GeroPsych* 23(4): 207–213.

Montgomery RJV, Gonyea JG and Hooyman NR. (1985) Caregiving and the experience of subjective and objective burden. *Family Relations* 34(1): 19–26.

Mu PF, Kuo HC and Chang KP. (2005) Boundary ambiguity, coping patterns and depression in mothers caring for children with epilepsy in Taiwan. *International Journal of Nursing Studies* 42: 273–282.

Muir CR and Haffey WJ. (1984) Psychological and neuropsychological interventions in the mobile mourning process. In: B. A. Edelstein and E. T. Couture (Eds.) *Behavioral Assessment and Rehabilitation of the Traumatically Brain Damaged*. New York: Plenum Press, pp. 247–272.

Murray CJL, Vos TL, Lozano R, Naghavi M, Flaxman AD, Michaud C, Ezzati M et al. (2010) Disability-adjusted years (DALYs) for 291 diseases and injuries in 21 regions, 1990–2010: A systematic analysis for the Global Burden of Disease Study 2010. *Lancet* 380: 2197–2223.

National Alliance for Caregiving and AARP. (2009) Caregiving in the United States 2009. www.caregiving.org/data/04finalreport.pdf (accessed 19 February 2014).

Nicholson NR. (2009) Social isolation in older adults: An evolutionary concept analysis. *Journal of Advanced Nursing* 65: 1342–1352.

Nicholson NR. (2012) A review of social isolation: An important but underassessed condition in older adults. *The Journal of Primary Prevention* 33(2–3): 137–152.

Nikfarid L, Rassouli M, Borimnejad L and Alavimajd H. (2015) Chronic sorrow in mothers of children with cancer. *Journal of Pediatric Oncology Nursing* 1–6.

North West Public Health Observatory. (2011) *Growing Older in Cumbria*. Liverpool, UK: North West Public Health Observatory.

Northington L. (2000) Chronic sorrow in caregivers of school age children with sickle cell disease: A grounded theory approach. *Issues in Comprehensive Pediatric Nursing* 23(3): 141–154.

Novi CD, Jacobs R and Migheli M. (2013) The quality of life of female informal caregivers: From Scandinavia to the Mediterranean Sea. CHE Research Paper 84. York, UK: University of York.

Noyes BB, Hill RD, Hicken BL, Luptak M, Rupper R, Dailey NK and Bair BD. (2010) The role of grief in dementia caregiving. *American of Alzheimer's Disease & Other Dementias* 25(1): 9–17.

O'Brien M. (2007) Ambiguous loss in families of children with autism spectrum disorder. *Family Relations* 56: 135–146.

Olshansky S. (1962) Chronic sorrow: A response to having a mentally defective child. *Social Casework* 43: 190–193.

Park CL. (1996) Stress-related growth and thriving through coping: The roles of personality and cognitive processes. *Journal of Social Issues* 54(2): 267–277.

Peacock S, Forbes D, Markle-Reid M, Hawranik P, Morgan D, Jansen L and Henderson SR. (2010) The positive aspects of the caregiving journey with dementia: Using a strengths-based perspective to reveal opportunities. *Journal of Applied Gerontology* 29: 640–659.

Pearlin LI, Mullan JT, Semple S and Skaff M M. (1990) Caregiving and the stress process: An overview of concepts and their measures. *The Gerontologist* 30(5): 583–594.

Peplau LA and Perlman D. (1982) Perspectives on loneliness. In: L. A. Peplau and D. Perlman (Eds.) *Loneliness: A Sources Book of Current Theory Research and Therapy.* New York: Wiley, pp. 1–8.

Phelps KW, Hodgson JL, McCammon SL and Lamson AL. (2009) Caring for an individual with autism disorder: A qualitative analysis. *Journal of Intellectual and Developmental Disability* 34(1): 27–35.

Picoraro JA, Womer JW, Kazak AE and Feudtner C. (2014) Posttraumatic growth in parents and paediatric patients. *Journal of Palliative Medicine* 17(2): 209–218.

Pinquart M and Sörensen S. (2003) Differences between caregivers and noncaregivers in psychological health and physical health: A meta-analysis. *Psychology and Aging* 18: 250–267.

Pinquart M and Sörensen S. (2005) Ethnic differences in stressors, resources, and psychological outcomes of family caregiving for older adults: A meta-analysis. *The Gerontologist* 45: 90–106.

Pinquart M and Sörensen S. (2006) Gender differences in caregiver stressors, social resources, and health: An updated meta-analysis. *Journal of Gerontology: Psychological Sciences* 61B: 33–45.

Pinquart M and Sörensen S. (2007) Correlates of physical health of informal caregivers: A meta-analysis. *Journal of Gerontology: Psychological Sciences* 62: 126–137.

Pinquart M and Sörensen S. (2011) Spouses, adult children, and children-in-law as caregivers of older adults: A meta-analytic comparison. *Psychology and Aging* 26(1): 1–14.

Prati G and Pietrantoni L. (2009) Optimism, social support, and coping strategies as factors contributing to posttraumatic growth: A meta-analysis. *Journal of Loss and Trauma* 14(5): 364–388.

Prigerson HG, Horowitz MG, Jacobs SC, Parkes CM, Aslan M, Goodkin K, Raphael B et al. (2009) Prolonged grief disorder: Psychometric validation of criteria proposed for DSM-V and ICD-11. *PLoS Medicine* 6: 1–12.

Rabins PV. (1984) Management of dementia in the family context. *Psychosomatics* 25: 369–375.

Rando TA. (Ed.) (1986) *Loss and Anticipatory Grief.* Lexington, MA: Lexington Books.

Rando TA. (2000) *Clinical Dimensions of Anticipatory Mourning: Theory Practice in Working with the Dying, Their Loved Ones and Their Caregivers.* Champaign, IL: Lexington Books.

Robinson B. (1983) Validation of the caregiver strain index. *Journal of Gerontology* 38: 344–348.

Roepke SK, Mausbach BT, Patterson TL, Von Känel R, Ancoli-Israel S, Harmell AL, Dimsdale JE, Aschbacher K, Mills PJ, Ziegler MG, Allison M, Grant I. (2011) Effects of Alzheimer caregiving on allostatic load. *Journal of Health Psychology* 16(1): 58–69.

Roick C, Heider D, Bebbington PE, Angermeyer MC, Azorin JM, Brugha TS, Kilian R, Johnson S, Toumi M, Kornfeld A, EuroSC Research Group. (2007) Burden on caregivers of people with schizophrenia: Comparison between Germany and Britain. *The British Journal of Psychiatry* 190: 333–338.

Rollins D, Waterman D and Esmay D. (1985) Married widowhood. *Activities, Adaptation and Aging* 7: 67–77.

Roos S. (2002) *Chronic Sorrow: A Living Loss*. New York: Brunner-Routledge.

Roper SO and Jackson JB. (2007) The ambiguities of out of-home care: Children with severe or profound disabilities. *Family Relations* 56: 147–161.

Rothman BK. (2000) *Recreating Motherhood*. 2nd edition. New Brunswick, NJ: Rutgers University Press.

Russell DW. (1996) UCLA loneliness scale (Version 3): Reliability, validity, and factor structure. *Journal of Personality Assessment* 66(1): 20–40.

Sanders S. (2005) Is the glass half empty or full? Reflections on strain and gain in caregivers of individuals with Alzheimer's disease. *Social Work in Health Care* 40: 57–73.

Sanders A and Szymanski K. (2013) Siblings of people diagnosed with a mental disorder and posttraumatic growth. *Community Mental Health Journal* 49(5): 554–555.

Sanders S and Adams KB. (2005) Grief reactions and depression in caregivers of individuals with Alzheimer's disease: Results from a pilot study in an urban setting. *Health & Social Work* 30(4): 287–295.

Sanders S, Ott CH, Kelber ST and Noonan P. (2008) The experience of high level of grief in caregivers of persons with Alzheimer's disease and related dementia. *Death Studies* 32(6): 496–523.

Schulz R and Beach SR. (1999) Caregiving as a risk factor for mortality: The caregiver health effects study. *Journal of the American Medical Association* 282(23): 2215–2219.

Shahly V, Chatterji S, Gruber MJ, Al-Hamzawi A, Alonso J, Andrade LH, Angermeyer MC et al. (2013) Cross-national difference in the prevalence and correlates of burden among older family caregivers in the WHO World Mental Health (WHM) surveys. *Psychological Medicine* 43(3): 865–879.

Skaff MM and Pearlin LI. (1992) Caregiving: Role engulfment and the loss of self. *The Gerontologist* 32(5): 656–664.

Smith GR, Williamson GM, Miller LS and Schulz R. (2011) Depression and quality of informal care: A longitudinal investigation of caregiving stressors. *Psychology and Aging* 26(3): 584–591.

Tedeschi RG and Calhoun LG. (1996) The posttraumatic growth inventory: Measuring the positive legacy of trauma. *Journal of Traumatic Stress* 9(5): 455–471.

Tedeschi RG and Calhoun LG. (2004) Posttraumatic growth: Conceptual foundations and empirical evidence. *Psychological Inquiry* 15(1): 1–18.

The Campaign to End Loneliness (CEL). (2011) Safeguarding the Convoy: A call to action from the Campaign to End Loneliness, Oxfordshire, UK. http://www.campaigntoendloneliness.org/ (accessed on May 2015).

The Children's Society. (2013) *Hidden from View: The Experiences of Young Carers in England*. London, UK: The Children's Society.

Theut SK, Jordan L, Ross LA and Deutsch SI. (1991) Caregiver's anticipatory grief in Dementia: A pilot study. *International Journal of Aging and Human Development* 33(2): 113–118.

Thrombre A, Sherman AC and Sinonton S. (2010) Religious coping and posttraumatic growth among family caregivers of cancers patients in India. *Journal of Psychosocial Oncology* 28: 178–188.

Travis SS, Bethea LS and Winn P. (2000) Medication administration hassles reported by caregivers of dependent elderly persons. *Journal of Gerontology: Medical Sciences* 55A(7): M412–M417.

United Nations. (2013) *World Population Aging 2013*. New York: United Nations.

Valizadeh L, Zamanzadeh V and Rahiminia E. (2013) Comparison of anticipatory grief reaction between fathers and mothers of premature infants in neonatal intensive care unit. *Scandinavian Journal of Caring Sciences* 27(4): 921–926.

Van Wijngaarden B, Schene A, Koeter M, Becker T, Knapp M, Knudsen HC, Tansella M et al. (2003) People with schizophrenia in five countries: Conceptual similarities and intercultural differences in family caregiving. *Schizophrenia Bulletin* 29: 573–586.

Viana MC, Gruber MJ, Shahly V, Alhamzawi A, Alonso J, Andrade LH, Angermeyer MC et al. (2013) Family burden related to mental and physical disorders in the world: Results from the WHO World Mental Health (WMH) surveys. *Revista Brasileira de Psiquiatria* 35(2): 115–125.

Vishnevsky T, Cann A, Calhoun LG, Tedeschi RG and Demakis GJ. (2010) Gender differences in self-reported posttraumatic growth: A meta-analysis. *Psychology of Women Quarterly* 34: 110–120.

Vitaliano PP, Zhang J and Scanlan JM. (2003) Is caregiving hazardous for one's physical health? A meta-analysis. *Psychological Bulletin* 129: 946–972.

Wadham O, Simpson J, Rust J and Murray C. (2015) Couples' shared experiences of dementia: A meta-synthesis of the impact upon relationships and couplehood. *Aging & Mental Health* 1–11. doi: 10.1080/13607863.2015.1023769.

Walker R, Pomeroy E, McNeil J and Franklin C. (1996) Anticipatory grief and AIDS: Strategies for intervening with caregivers. *Health and Social Work* 21(1): 49–58.

Walker RJ and Pomeroy EC. (1996) Depression or grief? The experience of caregivers of people with dementia. *Health & Social Work* 21: 247–254.

WHO. (1948) Preamble to the Constitution of the World Health Organization as adopted by the *International Health Conference*, New York, 19–22 June 1946, and entered into force on 7 April 1948.

Wilker LM, Wasow M and Hatfield E. (1981) Chronic sorrow revisited: Parents vs. professional depiction of the adjustment of parents of mentally retarded children. *American Journal of Orthopsychiatry* 51: 63–70.

World Federation of Mental Health (WFMH). (2010) Caring for the Caregiver: Why Your Mental Health Matters When You are Caring for Others. Woodbridge, VA: World Federation of Mental Health.

Wood RL and Yurdakul LK. (1997) Change in relationship status following traumatic brain injury. *Brain Injury* 11(7): 491–502.

Zamanzadeh V, Leila V, Elaheh R and Kochaksaraie FR. (2013) Anticipatory grief reactions in fathers of preterm infants hospitalized in neonatal intensive care unit. *Journal of Caring Sciences* 2(1): 83–88.

Zarit SH, Reever KE and Bach-Peterson J. (1980) Relatives of the impaired elderly: Correlates of feelings of burden. *The Gerontologist* 20(6): 649–655.

Zarit SH, Todd PA and Zarit JM. (1986) Subjective burden of husbands and wives as caregivers: A longitudinal study. *The Gerontologist* 26(3): 260–266.

Zarit SH. (2006) Caregivers assessment voices and views from the field. Report form *A National Consensus Development Conference*, Vol 11, Family Caregiver Alliance.

Zehner Ourada VE and Walker AJ. (2014) A comparison of physical health outcomes for caregiving parents and caregiving adult children. *Family Relations* 63(1): 163–177.

6

Providing Support and Interventions for Families and Carers

Introduction

This chapter begins with an overview of the assessment of family caregivers' needs and why this is important. This is followed by a discussion on the strategies for intervention, including individually focused, community-based services and support networks. The role of nurses in this process such as signposting and referral to various services and support groups is discussed. Finally, the importance of fostering hope in supporting families and carers is emphasised.

It is our intention in this chapter to provide insights into a range of interventions that can be used in practice to support family caregivers. Being able to offer practical solutions and suggestions is an essential attribute to 'being' a nurse. We appreciate that the 'doing' of nursing is important too, but in the context of supporting families and carers, the 'being' plays a significant part. We mention this distinction here as some interventions require the most fundamental of skills and subtleties such as those of listening, positive body language that transmit patience and time for hearing and listening alongside portraying that you have empathy, compassion and a caring attitude. Conversely, some of the interventions we will be discussing maybe less familiar to you, but that should not detract from their importance and value. Ultimately, the goal of any intervention is to avoid the development of secondary or hidden patients (caregivers).

As we have stated in the previous chapters, family caregivers embark upon the journey of caregiving often feeling thrust into uncharted territory of *being* a caregiver. As they navigate through their new role as a caregiver, they take on new responsibilities – face unforeseeable hardships and endure considerable challenges to their emotional and physical well-being. Healthcare professionals, notably nurses, have a pivotal role to play in helping family caregivers negotiate and navigate through these uncharted waters.

We believe that the benefits of using a salutogenic approach (focusing on health and positive aspects) can help to build health-promoting strategies for carers (see Chapter 4). We agree with Antonovsky (1979) that salutogenesis can help us understand health states and that there are some useful indicators that can be applied in practice. For example, it is through collaboration and partnership working that nurses can enable caregivers to understand their unique situation (compensability) and get involved in the process that enhances their health (manageability) so they can invest energy to solve problems (motivation/meaning). Thus, carers can be empowered and gain a sense of coherence. By understanding how carers manage their health and what resources they use, nurses can work with them to increase their ability to use positive resources. Further, as sense of coherence is developmental, it is important that nurses act early in the carer's life course or career in order to promote lifelong coping strategies and create positive mental health in preparation for their role.

The importance of identifying and supporting effective interventions that increase positive aspects and reduce negative aspects of caregiving has been the focus of many research studies. If nurses and other healthcare professionals are to improve the lives of family caregivers, then we need to take a holistic approach to providing support and interventions. Interventions applied to caregivers often have a theoretical framework, for example, the stress process model outlined in Chapter 3, which offers a means to understanding the effect of caregiving of a loved one, although the model does not include changing caregivers' behaviours. Changing caregivers' behaviours may require an approach that is underpinned by psychological theories that take into account the *whole family*, not just the caregiver and the care recipient. A systematic approach to the problems that caregivers face – burden of providing care and the associated stress and losses – is necessary if we are to improve the lives of family caregivers. Supporting families and carers is important for many reasons, including the following:

1. Families are the core of society, and supporting their ability to control and manage their situation increases their sense of liberty and independence.
2. Assisting families in functioning as a unit.
3. Supporting the family will also benefit care recipients.
4. Facilitating inclusion in society and enhancing their quality of life.
5. Assisting in mobilising families coping mechanisms and achieving affective and successful adaptation.

Assessment* of Families' and Caregivers' Needs

We know that caregiving can be extremely challenging and stressful for family caregivers, as we have seen in Chapter 5. Given that caregivers play an essential role in caring for their family members alongside the potential risks they can face in their tasks, their needs and capacities to provide care should be carefully and timely assessed as part of the holistic routine assessment process in regard of care planning.

Ideally, assessment should focus on the caregiver as both patient and provider before it can be assumed that the caregiver is able to provide competent care in the context of safe care for themselves or their family members. Unintentional harm may occur, for example, when a person with dementia is restrained in bed as a way to control wandering. By undertaking detailed assessments of the caregiving situation, through separate conversations with the patient and the caregiver, nurses may be able to identify these misguided practices or tasks and prevent abuse and neglect. Furthermore, holistic assessment in, and of, the home environment may also help to identify risk factors for unintentional harm and neglect and thus inform prevention processes to help reduce such harms. In addition, gathering information about how family caregivers have handled similar situations in the past is essential for problem-solving. By establishing what worked well in the past in dealing with adversity and what did not may also be useful in designing current interventions.

---

* Assessment in this context is not the Carers Assessment (UK Care Act 2014) as stated in Chapter 1 but assessment that is integral to nursing activity and care planning.

Nurses working in all areas of practice, especially in the community setting, are in pivotal positions to *get to know* the family and carer. In doing so, they are more likely to recognise caregiver strains and stressors and appropriately intervene to reduce the potential and actual negative impacts. Because of the heterogeneity of stressors, resources, values and other factors that affect the caregiving experience, individual caregiver assessment is fundamental. As the stress process model (see Chapter 3) advocates, primary and secondary stressors facing a particular family can vary considerably from each individual, and caregivers differ in what problems they find stressful. Also, caregivers respond to problems in different ways; for example, behaviours that most people would find upsetting, such as agitation or inappropriate language, may not hassle or overwhelm some caregivers, but for others, this may create immense distress. Thus, assessing what problems or challenges individual families find stressful is important in seeking assistance in relieving such stress. Furthermore, support should be tailored to individual preferences and needs. A holistic assessment also allows for the fostering of trust and therapeutic relationship between the nurse and the carer; opportunities in the community practice settings enable this process. A structured assessment of caregivers is important for several reasons, including the following:

1. Identifying clearly and precisely what problems are present in their situation
2. Clarifying the family's role and resources for caregiving, as well as the strains that care may be placing on their lives
3. Revealing that a family caregiver has urgent personal needs that need addressing
4. Identifying and determining eligibility for services that may be available
5. Providing evidence of needs as well as of the effectiveness of any interventions deployed to address the caregiver's problems
6. Relieving stress of family caregivers

A useful comprehensive model for assessing caregivers is provided by Given et al. (2012). Although this model is aimed at helping caregivers of people with cancer, we feel that this can be applied in the contexts of other caregivers as well. This model helps nurses to identify a caregiver's specific areas of needs and assist with selecting appropriate resources and interventions during their caregiving journey. The areas include the following:

- Caregiver's competing demands
- Living arrangements
- Caregiver's employment status
- Financial needs
- Demands in the level of care and time needed to provide that care
- Caregiver's knowledge and skills related to caregiving
- Caregiver's capacity and willingness to care
- Caregiver's own physical and mental health needs
- Available social and family resources
- Caregiver's expectations of the caregiving role

Thinking Box

Think of a family you have recently cared for.

What, how and when was an assessment performed?

Who undertook this assessment?

In reflecting back, do you think the model by Given et al. (2012) would have helped? In what ways?

Ongoing and Integral Assessment

There are many valid reasons to consider ongoing reassessments of family caregivers. First, caregiving is often a long-term commitment spanning many years. Changes in the care recipient's or caregiver's health may require amendments to the treatment plans or nature of support services. Furthermore, nurses cannot assume that a family carer is able to provide competent care without harming themselves or their family member; thus, nurses need to focus on the caregiver as both patient and provider. However, in the UK Care Act (2014), assessing carer's *ability* and *willingness* to care forms part of carers' assessment from April 2015 (see Chapter 1).

Ongoing integral (reassessment) also creates the opportunity to evaluate if planned interventions have achieved their intentions and goals and whether there are any new or unmet needs. Regular assessment may help to anticipate family caregivers' needs as they deal with myriad of problems that may be known to evolve over time. The frequency of reassessment will depend upon several factors, such as the dynamic nature of the health status of the patient and carer. Caring for those with long-term conditions is an enduring commitment and involves continually assessing the care recipient's needs as well as the carer's ability to meet the expected and, to some extent, unexpected needs.

Focused Assessments: Tools

The use of valid and reliable assessment tools can assist nurses and other healthcare professionals in focusing interventions on the needs of family caregivers. Assessment tools are commonly used to identify problems that then can be targeted for appropriate and timely interventions. Many tools exist especially in the field of dementia care. Specific assessment tools address areas such as burden and depression, e.g., hospital and anxiety depression scale, and others are readily available, easy to administer and both reliable and valid. Some of these have already been highlighted throughout this book. Further, the assessment of family caregivers' coping aptitude and burden is useful to guide nurses and other healthcare professionals in planning for respite care and/or other support services that may be needed. Early recognition of the negative impact of caregiving is beneficial in preventing the onset of major health problems for caregivers and any adverse effects in connection to their loved ones.

Undoubtedly, the nurse is best placed to explore through direct questioning key aspects related to family and friends support networks and any feelings of isolation such as 'where do other family members live?' and 'how often do they see them?' It is equally important to establish if these relationships are positive ones, as divergent or strained relationships may place additional demands on the carer and be potentially detrimental to their health. Seeking to obtain information about family and friends is an important aspect in discharge planning from hospital, in particular for considering support networks and practical help that is likely to be available (or not).

Following the assessment of those who are deemed vulnerable of becoming socially isolated and those who may require assistance with social integration, they can be referred to community resources such as signposting to carers' centres or information resources, websites and social networking tools. Future visits and assessments by the community nurse or specialist nurses should focus on developing agreed plans of care that reduce and prevent social isolation.

It may be necessary to observe and question the caregiver regarding any manifestation of grief, which may include unusual physical symptoms or feeling excessively sad, angry, helpless, guilty or anxious; any appetite or sleep disturbances; or difficulty in concentrating. In addition, it is important to determine the key points on when changes in the care recipient or *mini-deaths* may create intense feeling of loss (Marwit and Meuser 2005), along with previous losses, and what coping strategies the caregiver may have used so as to capitalise on adaptive coping and support for those in need of help.

Key Points

- The needs of the carer should be assessed holistically.
- Assessment of caregiver should be ongoing and integral.
- Assessments may include focused assessments using validated tools.

Interventions to Support Families and Carers

Interventions to facilitate family coping often utilise aspects of the various stress models, as discussed in Chapter 3, to help families regain a pre-crisis equilibrium. The literature provides substantial evidence that caregivers are *hidden patients* and thus are in need of protection from physical and emotional impairment and warrant guidance and safeguarding. The interventions that a nurse can provide in supporting families and carers need to be flexible and individualistic. However, there are some general principles that may be applicable in all situations and those include providing information and education, helping to manage stressors and providing emotional and instrumental support. Working in partnership with families and caregivers, nurses are in key positions both in acute hospital setting and in community to provide this support. Nurses should be concerned with several issues that affect patient safety and quality of care as the reliance and dependency on family caregiving grows. Whatever the interventions, the fact that nurses and family caregivers are partners in healthcare and carers need to be engaged throughout every aspect of care planning should be recognised. This is critical for those with long-term conditions/chronic illnesses. In addition, the differences in caregiving, regarding gender and coping, ought to be accounted for in planning interventions to support caregivers. Due to the fact that coping is amenable to fluctuation and deviations in response to interventions, discovering coping strategies in family caregivers is an important endeavour.

Interventions directed at the family caregiver have two main purposes. First, interventions can support the family caregiver as *a patient* directly reducing the adverse impact of caregiving on their health and well-being, as seen in Chapter 5. This support enables caregivers to continue to bear the physical, social and financial costs of their caregiving responsibilities. Of course, such interventions, whilst directed at caregivers by implication, benefit the care recipient (patient), i.e., if we alleviate the suffering in the non-injured (the family carer), then we help the injured (the patient). Second, interventions are used to increase caregiver's competence and confidence in providing safe and effective care to their family member. As family caregivers are unpaid providers, they often need specific assistance to understand and attain knowledge to become competent and safe in their roles so as to protect their family members (i.e. the care recipients) from harm. This may also indirectly affect caregivers by reducing their burden or distress and increasing their sense of control, certainty and mastery.

For those carers who combine their caring responsibilities with paid work, interventions may be necessary to help support carers balance their dual responsibilities. The wider implication of this has been highlighted in a recent UK report 'Supporting Working Carers' (Carers UK 2013) that makes recommendations for supporting carers to combine work with caregiving. According to Carers UK (2013), one-third of carers reported that they had given up paid work or reduced their working hours because support services were inadequate or too expensive. The suggestion here is that with adequate support these carers may be supported to remain in employment and balance their dual roles. As we have stated, with the growth of societies' ageing population (UN 2013; WHO 2014), the number of carers leaving the workforce will also increase, which is detrimental to both the wider community and the economy of a country.

Individually Focused Support

Individually focused interventions that seek to ensure that caregivers (particularly in the home and community setting) can perform their roles can, broadly speaking, be divided into four main areas:

1. Informational – information about care, quality of life, prognoses, symptoms, injuries, diseases, sequelae and implications
2. Emotional – listening, caring and respecting
3. Practical – decision-making, counselling services and encouraging family members to participate
4. Financial

Providing Appropriate Information

Nurses need to communicate effectively with patients and caregivers to develop effective care planning and achieve positive outcomes. Communication is crucial in all interactions with patients and their caregivers. At all points in a patient's disease trajectory, caregivers need information to deal with the patient's care and treatment demands. Caregivers require knowledge, skills and judgement to carry out the tasks of caring for their loved ones, and research has shown that caregivers who feel prepared to deliver care (i.e. have the knowledge and skills needed) have less burden (Scherbring 2002). Nurses and other healthcare professionals should not expect caregivers to be responsible for *sorting out* relevant information aligned to their situation and making sense of it. Crucially, nurses ought to understand/appreciate the information and support the needs of caregivers they are engaging with. The goal here is to establish a sense of people's health literacy and capacity to understand the body of information available so as to tailor individual support for carers in their roles and contexts. Providing appropriate and timely information along with emotional support can help caregivers better manage their caregiving situation. Providing information in a variety of modes – verbal, written and electronic – needs to be considered. In addition, nurses can pre-empt information needs as part of future planning and long-term needs. Anticipatory planning here can help to relieve caregivers' distress arising from uncertainties about their family members' disease or illness, treatments and therapies they may need. The alternative is that uncertainty due to lack of information gives a feeling of helplessness and loss of situational control (Plowfield 1999). As noted by Lazarus and Folkman (1984), lack of information plays a significant role in creating overload or *pile-up* (see Chapter 3).

Providing effective education and information at the right time and place is instrumental in promoting and providing a foundation for certainty. Anticipating circumstances when uncertainty may be increased, i.e., changes in a loved one's condition, can be supported by nurses referring to specialists for additional supportive information, although some information may increase anxiety and disrupt feelings of hope. Hence, getting information may be a constant worry, adding to the carer's stress, which may involve considerable effort to find someone to ask for information.

There is no getting away from the fact that providing information can be challenging, not least because information-seeking behaviours are highly individualistic. Nurses need to be sensitive to the carers' information needs and level of health literacy. Too much information too soon can be overwhelming and may not be retained, and too little or too late information can undermine confidence in the healthcare professionals and the family member's sense of control and ability to plan. Signposting caregiver to useful resources throughout the disease trajectory is important because caregivers are often unaware of support services available to them. Providing local intelligence as to where to access information and supportive help about resources and services such as respite enables carers to make informed knowledge-based decisions about their loved ones.

As we have suggested, families' information needs vary notably on a day-to-day basis as in the context of a critical care setting. In the critical care environment, families need information about their loved one's condition, progress and prognosis. When a family member is hospitalised, nurses need to provide information to the family members about the daily care of their loved one, the environment (ward/unit), any relevant equipment and what they can do for the patient during the visit times. Family members want information on the condition and the treatment of the patient and that information needs to reassure them that the best care is being provided.

Thinking Box

Can you think back to an example in practice of giving information to a family caregiver, what helped?

In reflecting back, could these have been done differently? And in what ways could these have been improved?

Emotional and Instrumental Support

Emotional and instrumental support may be available from family and friends. However, caregivers may become isolated from their networks as a result of their caregiving responsibilities. Nurses are in key positions to provide both emotional support and inform and train caregivers in new skills. However, this needs to be carried out in the context of a supportive, non-judgemental relationship. Within the safety of this relationship, caregivers may be able to explore alternatives, i.e. learn new skills, try new approaches and behaviours and develop a better understanding of their situation. This can ultimately result in improved outcomes for both the patient and the carers themselves. Furthermore, interventions that help family caregivers appraise their situations differently, i.e., more positively, could result in an increased sense of meaning. Of note here, Quinn et al. (2010, 2012) show that increasing or improving caregiver's competences and skills results in an increased sense of meaning. A supportive relationship that enables a sense of meaning has scope to benefit the triad relationship between carer, nurse and care recipient, one that respects and values each other's roles and skills in caring. By fostering ways to offer emotional and instrumental support, nurses can significantly impact on the lives of carers and their families.

Interventions to Support Loss

One of the first steps in helping caregivers to cope with their grief is recognising their grief responses. Many caregivers do not understand that what they are experiencing is normal. Providing information on the grieving process and on the nature of anticipatory mourning can directly relieve unnecessary suffering. However, if this grief becomes complicated, then the nurse should be able to identify this situation so that appropriate referrals can be instigated. Although some research indicated that anticipatory grief does have a positive adaptive effect by easing the intensity of grief for the bereaved after the actual death, others have indicated that caregivers are more likely to require bereavement services. Understanding the impact of chronic sorrow and being aware of trigger events that may cause a period of sadness can be helpful in contingency planning so as to help family members accept that such responses are normal. The primary goals for nurses in managing chronic sorrow are directly linked to recognising and allowing the person to express their feelings. Recognising that chronic sorrow is a natural reaction to ongoing losses is an important starting point. Equally, labelling the experience of ambiguous loss for caregivers is important, for, in most cases, caregivers are not aware that their distress, confusion and immobility are located in their inherently ambiguous situation and not in themselves. Boss (1999, 2004, 2006) clearly conveys that identifying the source of the difficulty in the loss that people have experienced can be a major step towards helping individuals reorganise their thinking. Thus, in doing so, they can begin to employ their usual coping mechanisms rather than remaining 'stuck' in a pattern that is no longer appropriate to their changed family circumstances.

In chronic sorrow, facilitating families to adapt to their losses, supporting them emotionally during recurring periods of sadness and validating their feelings of loss are critical. Nurses can provide supportive care by developing a therapeutic relationship with family members such as by spending time to listen to them, respecting their individuality as a family member and allowing expressions of sadness. In addition, providing positive feedback on how the caregivers are coping in times of sadness has been found to be a useful approach by healthcare professionals in coping with chronic sorrow (Damrosch and Perry 1989).

Nurses need to take time to understand how a person comprehends their losses and assist them in making their loss experience more manageable (Rando 2000). Providing a 'listening ear', so that family caregivers can express their feelings, may be the only intervention required, but over time more help may be needed; in such instances, referrals to bereavement counsellors or caregiver support groups would help. Research has demonstrated that the experience of anticipatory mourning in caregivers strongly indicates the necessity to include bereavement and other support services before and after the death of a loved one due to protracted illness (Johansson and Grimby 2011). Furthermore, Johansson and Grimby (2011) also posit that the identification of anticipatory grief, at the very early stages of the caregiving trajectory, could pave the way for the development of strategies that better support caregivers' well-being and can maximise their ability to aid their family member as the family member's health status declines. If nurses are to support those adaptive coping strategies of families and inspire hope, they need to understand the families' losses.

Journaling

Relatives and family members can find it very useful on many levels to keep a journal or diary to note down their experiences and/or the journey of their loved ones (Jacelon and Imperio 2005). It can be a cathartic experience and a valuable resource for some families.

Journaling offers for some family caregivers the opportunity to cognitively organise stressful events and provides an avenue for reflection on their often overwhelming and difficult daily lives. There is no right or wrong way to journal; it simply involves writing whatever comes to mind. Pennebaker's (1997, 1999) research found a link between the therapeutic effects of journal writing about personally upsetting experiences on one's well-being. This is later supported by the work of Jacelon and Imperio (2005) who state that journal writing promotes focus on daily activities and reflections that people value. Indeed, in the context of critical illness (e.g. visiting in critical care environments), journals and diaries can play a positive role in the quality of life of, and recovery for, close relatives or family members, although according to Agard and Lomborg (2010), we need to know more about the overall impact of acute and critical illnesses on both patients and relatives. As we know, this is a time of great uncertainty for all involved, notably the close family and friends. Therefore, seeking to find meaning and understanding and making sense of what has happened during a critical and/or unexpected illness and the subsequent aftermath is challenging for most people. With this in mind, it is perceived that diary/journal accounts may be of help in long-term recovery of critical ill survivors and their close relatives. Moreover, by going over their past journal entries, caregivers can trace their growth and development, which may increase their problem-solving skills and be a source of hope for the future.

Blogging

Blogging, evolving as an online communication space, gives voice to feelings and expressions that can help people to cope, adapt to their circumstance or just enable them to 'speak out' or 'vent off'. Blogging serves as a medium of support for both the author and readers of the blog. It has been suggested that writing and reading of blogs enables like-minded people (Papacharissi 2004) to gain agency, build social capital (Chung and Kim 2007) and share their *minority*, or otherwise, views. This can be really useful to carers and their loved ones, and the potential to connect with like-minded people is huge. Like journals and diaries, the words written in a blog have therapeutic benefits, and by nature of being accessible these offer possibilities for engagement with others. Ure (2015), in his small survey on breast cancer survivors' blogs, found that breast cancer survivors benefitted from blogging, as a way to challenge current UK media representations of breast cancer *survivorship* and post-treatment issues. Clearly, other social media also play a role in supporting ongoing psychosocial needs. It is not within the scope of this book to explore social media in any detail, but at this juncture it is worth acknowledging that this is an area that is developing rapidly. For example, most charities dedicated to supporting carers have their own Twitter accounts, and they use hashtags, '#', to theme discussions pertinent to carers and families. Individual carers are visible and active on Twitter concerning ways either to promote their views, ideas and current issues or to raise awareness of carer's existence, contributions and roles. Of course, the context of social media means that variations in between these two positions exist.

Educating Family Carers

An important starting point prior to implementing any interventions with caregivers is identifying what knowledge and understanding they possess about their family members' illness, implications of that illness and the long-term options for care. Often at the point when caregivers seek assistance, they have very little information, and finding ways to educate caregivers will help them understand what they should not do and why they need help.

When caring for someone with dementia or other mental health problems, caregivers may misinterpret behaviours which may lead to increased stress for both themselves and their loved ones. For example, caregivers may believe that their relative with cognitive impairment who repeatedly asks the same questions may be doing so to annoy or aggravate them. This may lead the caregiver to respond with anger or exasperation, which in turn only increases the patient's agitation. This may further aggravate the caregiver's anger and frustration, thus making the situation critical. Community nurses are in key positions to teach families about their relatives' condition and help them to interpret challenging behaviours as part of the disease process or condition in order for them to gain a better understanding of their situation. For example, teaching caregivers how to manage pain and other symptoms can benefit both the patient and caregiver. Nurses also play a critical role in teaching and educating caregivers in the use of medical equipment in support of their loved ones, such as home oxygen therapy.

As a result of many years of caregiving, caregivers build up high level of expertise, skill and tacit knowledge. Family members are central to providing daily tasks, direct and indirect, for patients with long-term conditions. This may involve medical equipment such as home oxygen, complex medication regimes and treatments for symptom control. This expertise and tacit knowledge are particularly important in decision-making during symptom exacerbations, for example, in chronic obstructive disease or congestive heart disease. As the basis for educational interventions and collaborative learning, shared decision-making should be promoted within the context of the triad relationship between carer, nurse and care recipient.

Key Points

- Interventions to support families and carers are integral to holistic nursing care and enhance salutogenesis.
- Provision of information alone is not enough, and information interventions need to be focused and individually tailored.
- Interventions that deal with loss, grief and coping require time to listen and understand.

Developing Family Caregivers' Problem-Solving Skills

Nurses can play a role in helping caregivers to develop and address their problem-solving skills. Of course, carers are faced with many problems on a day-to-day basis. Family caregivers may face many problems associated with their role, for example, problems associated with adhering to complex medical tasks and ensuring their loved one adheres to therapeutic regimens. Problem-solving can be defined as a self-directed process aimed at identifying solutions for specific problems encountered in daily life (D'Zurilla and Nezu 2007). A collaborative, problem-solving approach can generate practical solutions for addressing problems and challenges that carers face. Through discussion and active listening to the caregiver, alternative realistic approaches for managing the situation or a particular issue can be explored. For instance, a particular service may be inadequate or the caregiver may be reluctant to accept help due to uncertainty, lack of confidence or a belief that they should provide all the care for their loved ones. Many of the daily challenges of caregiving can be relieved through systematic examination of the caregiver's antecedents that trigger problem behaviour such as agitation and the consequences that reinforce the behaviour. By helping to identify patterns of antecedents and consequences, the nurses and carers can identify possible solutions. Caring for a person with cognitive impairment, such as

Alzheimer's disease or brain injury, may include changing environment cues that trigger a problematic behaviour. It must also be recognised that caregivers may need time to consider alternative options. In some circumstances, the shared decision-making process may be very delicate and complex, for example, ceasing to care and placing their loved ones into a residential care or a nursing home.

Interestingly, D'Zurilla and Nezu (2007) propose a problem-solving intervention that nurses may find useful, which resonates with problem-solving approaches inherent within the nursing process which encourages individuals to modify their thinking about stressors and address problems using five related steps: attitude, define, alternatives, predict and try out (ADAPT). Before the carer can embark on this process, the carer needs to be encouraged to adopt an optimistic attitude towards their ability to effectively solve problems. Problem-solving is the process by which an individual copes with a problem by attempting to adapt solutions to a given event or situation. More specifically, problem-solving reflects a person's ability to rationally apply four problem-solving skills: defining a problem, generating alternative solutions, deciding on a solution and implementing and evaluating the solution plan. The ability to solve problems and make decisions is an important aspect of the caregiving role. The skill of problem-solving, however, is highly influenced by negative emotions (anxiety, stress, anger, fear and depression), and as caregivers are often faced with a situation to take complex decisions, problem-solving skills play a major role. The basis of problem-solving skills is that the use of a constructive problem-solving style enables the caregiver to possess skills and beliefs that help them to regulate their emotions, maintain a positive attitude (for solving problems) and use rational, instrumental and problem-solving strategies. In contrast, a carer using ineffective problem-solving skills typically relies on impulsive, thoughtless, careless and ineffective methods to solve problems.

Enhancing problem-solving abilities can be useful in helping and supporting caregivers through difficult problems and situations by talking through the specific problems with them and offering effective solutions or ways of coping. Results from several studies, across diverse conditions, demonstrate the effectiveness of problem-solving training in lowering depressive symptoms and burden and increasing the well-being experienced by family caregivers of children with brain injuries (Wade et al. 2006; Rivera et al. 2008), stroke survivors (Lui et al. 2005) people with spinal cord injuries (Elliott et al. 2008; Elliott and Berry 2009) and people with severe disabilities (Elliot et al. 2009; Berry et al. 2012). In essence, obtaining a solution to a problem is considered as specific response to the problem, and an effective solution achieves the goal of changing the situation and reducing the negative emotions. Perhaps in practice it is not that simple, but we do know that the therapeutic nature of being able to talk and listen can serve as a huge step forward.

Perhaps, rather more complex is the experience of loss in caregivers, where particular high levels of anticipatory grief, and this has been associated with a diminished ability to solve problems (Fowler et al. 2013). Other researches have found that depression and decreased life satisfaction of the caregiver significantly affect their problem-solving abilities (Bambara et al. 2009). This has the potential to cause more problems in the caregiving role as they are faced with challenging situations and complexities that can impact problem-solving. Both Fowler et al. (2013) and Bambara et al. (2009) highlight that ineffective problem-solving abilities account for more variance in the prediction of caregiver depression than other demographic variables amongst caregivers. Thus, enhancing problem-solving skills is an important intervention for nurses and other healthcare professionals to be concerned about and prioritised.

Community-Focused Support and Services

Support Groups

Support groups are a popular intervention for family caregivers. Historically, they arose in response to caregivers' feeling that their information and help needs were not being met by healthcare professionals. Generally, support groups consist of regular face-to-face group meetings that are time limited and often structured. Of course support groups vary in their structure; for example, some provide drop-in sessions with modest hospitality (e.g. cups of tea), whilst others provide more structured formats with external speakers invited to talk about specific topics. The premise of any support group is to learn from and to support one another. Research evidence indicates that they can provide emotional support and information and improve carers' problem-solving skills. Generally, they serve to provide practical information to caregivers and particularly different ways of coping with the consequences of their caregiving role. Caregivers can share information with other caregivers about what works for them and what they found helpful along with possible practical suggestions. Attendance may also help caregivers to manage difficult or challenging issues and even offer respite. Support groups can, for some caregivers, be a safe and practical way of sharing their feelings and thoughts with like-minded people who have experienced similar issues, i.e., a sense of 'walking in their shoes'. For some caregivers, social support is an important interactive process providing emotional support, as connecting with others may help to reduce fears and uncertainty and validate their experiences so that they realise that they are not alone. In addition to support groups which are long established in many communities, multifamily groups (MFGs) and peer support programmes are emerging as other avenues to support family caregivers. Evidence suggests, from a variety of carer populations, that MFGs are effective interventions in improving family functioning and well-being and that they bring families together.

However, there may be a reluctance to use such support groups for a variety of realistic and unrealistic reasons, i.e., the belief that it is wrong to seek help and that it is one's duty or obligation to care. Undoubtedly, family caregivers who are in paid work may have limited opportunity in terms of time to physically attend support groups and engage in community support opportunities. In such instances, community support that can be tailored to individual needs can be helpful; e.g., carer support centre offering evening sessions and drop-in, one-to-one appointments with professionals. It can be here that social media or blogging can serve to support local people in a virtual world rather than in a physical sense.

Whilst the evidence is limited on effective interventions for addressing isolation in caregiving, there is a substantial body of evidence that has reviewed the effectiveness of interventions for decreasing social isolation. Although most studies included in these reviews focus on the older person, the interventions that appear to be the most effective include regular social group activities/programmes and support interventions, such as counselling therapy, training on Internet use and education (Cattan et al. 2005; Dickens et al. 2011; Masi et al. 2011).

In terms of community nursing engagement with families and carers, continuity of care has been shown to be an effective intervention, for example, in reducing social isolation and in improving health outcomes and the sense of meaning and belonging. In response to a large-scale 2014 carers' project funded by the UK Department of Health, The Queen's Nursing Institute (QNI) developed three free online resources to support nurses who work with carers. The QNI's commitment to carers is ongoing and strong, with numerous useful resources are available on their website; see http://www.qni.org.uk/supporting_carers. However, caring for carers is an integral and explicit dimension of nursing practice, whatever the setting.

Respite Care

Respite care is often considered a fundamental support provision for carers with the recognised benefit of reducing caregiver burden and stress. The temporary relief from their caregiving responsibilities is often described as a 'breather break' and is a chance to step back and recuperate. Respite may be for a short or long period of time and can be for the carer and/or care recipient. Care recipient's adult day care in general as a structured, community-based comprehensive programme provides a variety of health, social and related support services for specific periods of time, whereas day-care services depend upon the needs of the caregivers or more domiciliary respite in which relief is provided by healthcare professionals. These services provide an opportunity for the social interaction and important peer support for the caregiver. However, there may be issues of transportation, for those carers in rural areas, to and from day centres. Carer charities can offer carer respite through personal budgets in collaboration with local authorities, although such provision varies across the United Kingdom. Examples of respite care in this context can be carer day trips, social events or one-off purchases of low-cost resources as a means of offering respite in a person's own home such as a laptop or garden shed.

Long-term respite care includes residential respite care such as in nursing homes, residential care homes and hospitals that provide respite services. Evidence suggests that caregivers may be reluctant to use these services because of cost, transportation, inflexible hours and feelings of resentment towards the service providers (Kosloski and Montgomery 1995; Cox 1997). Limited availability and cost implications, however, raise the issue of helping families find appropriate provision that meets the needs and expectations of both the caregiver and care receivers. Nurses, through signposting, can help carers navigate the available services that best meets their needs. However, strong beliefs in family obligation and privacy may dissuade caregivers and care recipients to access community provision and see it as a *last resort* or only in cases when they are desperate, i.e., at the 'end of the road', rather than a preventative or supportive opportunity. Some family caregivers may find notions of *letting go* or *handing over* care responsibilities to others difficult, and negative beliefs about services can be strong influencing factors for declining respite possibilities. With this mindset, when they finally come to use these services, they may feel that community services accessed may be insufficient or inadequate in meeting their needs. Consequently, this outcome may increase their frustration and sense of hopelessness alongside their emotional strain. If carers find that the respite provision does not meet their expectations, then they are more likely to be reluctant to seek access and use such services in the future. Cultural influences may also play an important role in respite desires and decision-making processes. Of note, the concept of familism and heteronormativity can influence perceptions of respite access and experiences. Irrespective of family structure or features, the use of respite services has been shown to reduce caregiver's accounts of role captivity (feeling of being trapped and having no choice in their role) (Gaugler et al. 2003).

Of course, it is clear that the decision to seek and untimely use respite services is a complex one. Several factors have been identified that may contribute to the caregivers' perception of the unmet need of their loved ones and dissatisfaction with the service, including service availability, service sufficiency, service adequacy, cultural *norms* and sensitivity of services, time schedules of the services and control over who provides the service. Families also need to be confident and trust that respite will fulfil their loved one's needs and expectations. Trust is an influencing factor as carers need to feel that their loved one is in 'safe hands'. Phillipson et al. (2013) in an Australian study of carers of people with dementia reported that carers' believed that respite services would result in negative outcomes for their loved ones, which was strongly associated with non-use of respite services. Similarly, Stirling et al. (2014) report that carers needed to trust that their loved ones would receive quality experience and meet their perceived expectations in order for them to take up respite care.

Alternatively, respite in one's own home may occur on a regular or occasionally and can take place in a more flexible manner (during the day, evenings, at weekends). In-home respite may be more acceptable to some family caregivers as they can remain in the comfort of their own environment and have no transportation issues. In this context, options can be through voluntary sector as well as official services. However, some families may be reluctant to use in-home respite services due to being uncomfortable or fearful of having *strangers* in their homes engaging with their loved ones.

Technological/Assistive Technology Interventions

More innovative ways of providing community support and addressing the underutilisation of the services that are available are possible today through information technologies. Telehealth telecare and assistive information and communications technology (ICT) solutions play a significant part in supporting caregivers in numerous ways. Telehealth programmes can be delivered by synchronous technology (e.g. telephone call, video conferencing and instant messaging) which permits real-time connections between the family carer and nurse, or asynchronous technology (e.g. self-guided web exercises, discussion boards and email) where information is stored or sent and then retrieved at a later point in time. Of course, some programmes use a combination of such modes.

Carers UK suggest that telehealth and technologies enable carers to combine work and caregiving. Carers who manage physical distances or multiple care responsibilities, such as sandwich carers, distance carers and young carers, may find these interventions particularly useful. Increasingly, technological products and resources are becoming available to support carers and families to assist in managing their busy and complex lives. The UK incentives such as the Technology-Enabled Care Services (TECS) programme at NHS England aims to provide resources and practical tools for health and social care workers to support, guide and evaluate such technological solutions and services. Whilst in the European Union, a recent report on the provision of household and personal services identifies ICT support as one of the broad range of services that contribute to the well-being of families and individuals (Farvaque 2013).

Telehealth, due to its accessibility, convenience and potentiality to be user friendly, can be a useful intervention across the age range. Assumptions by age should not be made for example, older carers can be very eager to use telehealth. Telehealth has scope to be used in training, learning and providing information. In addition, providing problem-solving skills training via telephone has been shown to be successful with family caregivers of stroke survivors after rehabilitation (Grant et al. 2002), and similar outcomes have been observed for training via the Internet (Wade et al. 2006). The benefits of this approach are increased access for families in rural areas as well as reduced costs of transportation. For those family members requiring specialist services which cover large geographical areas, this method may be particularly beneficial. Internet use has been shown to contribute to older adults' feelings of well-being. Telephone consultations for caregivers residing in the community may reinforce the sense of partnership between the healthcare professional and the carer. It may also circumvent any issues or challenges that the carer may face and reduce the potential for a crisis.

Befriending and Community Navigators (Practical Solution Community/Individual)

In helping to combat social isolation in the United Kingdom, a report by Social Care Institute for Excellence (Windle et al. 2011) provides some useful practical interventions to address social isolation or loneliness, for example, one-to-one interventions such as befriending, Community Navigators, group meetings and wider community engagement. Befriending is defined as 'an intervention that introduces the client to one or more individuals, whose main aim is to provide the client with additional social support through the development of an affirming, emotion-focused relationship over time' (Mead et al. 2010, p. 96). There are a variety of befriending models ranging from regular face-to-face contact (visiting an individual in their own home) to regular telephone contact and group meetings and they usually involve volunteers or paid workers from the community. This intervention has been found to reduce loneliness and social isolation following the intervention and is valued by service users (Mentoring and Befriending Foundation [MBF] 2010). Many of the befriending schemes have emerged at the community level to 'fill the social and emotional gap that is seemingly unmet by existing statutory health and social service provision' (Mentoring and Befriending Foundation [MBF] 2010). Community Navigators provide hard-to-reach or vulnerable people with emotional, practical and social support (Windle et al. 2011). Compared to *usual care*, Knapp et al. (2010) found that befriending interventions and Community Navigator schemes were cost effective. Both befriending and Community Navigators are important in providing companionship and a sense of belonging that resonate with a sense of worth and inclusion.

Interestingly, the Marmot Review (2010) that examined and proposed a new way to reduce health inequalities in England post-2010 recognised the value of social networks in maintaining and improving health and well-being. Marmot recommended that locally developed and evidence-based community regeneration programmes that reduce social isolation should be maintained and supported. Similarly, in a review by Knapp et al. (2010), the importance of building community capacity to help alleviate problems such as loneliness was highlighted. In nursing practice, and especially health visiting, it is known that community development has capacity to tackle the effects of poverty and social deprivation and as such can play an important role in tackling loneliness (Lauder et al. 2006).

Thinking Box

Have you come across such schemes in practice?

If not, perhaps seek out local schemes and make contact so as to be able to recommend to families and carers.

Fostering Hope

On the one hand, hope is recognised as an important aspect of coping, dealing with adversity and an essential element for carer's resilience, yet it has received limited attention in the caregiving literature. Hope inspirations and hope promotion are vital assets to a nurse and are part of the caring/empathetic and trust qualities of nursing. Given that hope fluctuates in an individual's life, notably during caregiving, it can decrease and be challenged amongst families and caregivers; nurses are in a key position to maintain and foster hope.

Fostering hope is multidirectional in that strategies that are supportive of maintaining hope in families can also indirectly affect the care recipient. Equally, fostering hope in care recipients can inspire hope in their close families and carers. This emphasises that although inspiring hope in caregivers may depend on nurses and other healthcare professionals, care recipients also play a part in the process of fostering hope in families. The literature is scant on the influence of hope on caregiving and in particular the role of facilitating and fostering hope in supporting families and caregivers. Whilst the literature makes a case for the need to develop hope-enhancing interventions, their effectiveness has not been adequately examined. Principles based on the hope models discussed in Chapter 4 can be applied by nurses to family caregivers for maintaining and fostering hope.

Hope may arise within moments when fear, hopelessness or despair seems just as likely. When family caregiver's hopes are unrealistic in that their goals appear unattainable and are rooted in the past, hope can be hindered. False hopes serve to prevent carers from seeking solutions and information. Nurses can help family caregivers to stimulate and develop their rediscovery of hope. This arguably starts by having a physical presence within the family, validating and empathising with their experiences in an attempt to understand their situation and needs by keeping them appraised of their situation. Attending to families and caregivers and listening and asking questions combined with building trust undoubtedly help to develop a therapeutic relationship between the family and nurse (i.e. a triad relationship). However, this is reliant upon certain key intangible attributes of the nurse, including open communication, compassion, concern, commitment and respect. One of the few studies by Turner and Stokes (2006) exploring nurse's use of patient hope-promoting strategies found that nurses had limited understanding or knowledge of hope strategies. Several qualitative studies of hope in a variety of patient groups, including the critically ill, older adults and the terminally ill, have identified potential hope-promoting strategies, such as defining and refocusing goals and aims and cognitive strategies (e.g. reappraising the situation), facilitating the expression of spiritual beliefs and practices (Herth 2001). Threats to hope have also been identified, including lack of information, isolation, fatigue and sleep deprivation and losses associated with caregiving, such as anticipatory grief and ambiguous loss, as described in Chapter 5. Thus, nurses need to have knowledge of hope-promoting and hope threat–reducing strategies as both are important to the family and their loved one.

Thinking Box

Think about your current practice. Do you believe that having and conveying hope is important?

What hopes and expectations do you have for a family and/or carer you are caring for? And do these resonate with those of the family or caregivers?

What specific hope strategies have you used to inspire hope with family caregivers?

Interestingly, Miller (1991) proposed several categories of hope inspiration for families of the critically ill, including expanding families' coping repertoire, finding meaning in the illness/situation, focusing on a generalised hope state, reducing uncertainty regarding care, using presence and humour, maximising hope contagion, eliminating cognitive distortion and sustaining caring therapeutic relationships. In line with Snyder's goal-orientated hope theory (1994, 2000) (discussed in Chapter 4), families have a tendency to feel hopeful when goals are clear and their pathway is known. Hopelessness unfolds when the pathway feels blocked or when the goal is unknown. Therefore, helping carers to clarify their goals and pathways is very helpful in the quest to develop and maintain hope. Statements by caregivers such as 'I can do this' and 'I can find a way' may highlight those who are more hopeful and able to pursue their goals despite obstacles. Thus, by identifying personally meaningful and plausible goals, exploring ways to break them down to manageable steps and helping carers to be prepared to be flexible with setbacks or obstacles, nurses can foster hope in family carers.

One of the major concerns of all family members is obtaining truthful and comprehensive information that permits the creation of realistic hope (Verhaeghe et al. 2007a,b). Thus, the pursuit of realistic hope relies heavily upon information that is understandable, accurate and thorough. For some caregivers, information seeking to secure control in personal decision-making serves as a major coping strategy. Verhaeghe et al. (2007a,b) revealed, in their study of family, that all family members have a need for hope and that concrete hope seems to be strongly determined by adequate information. In addition, providing a supportive environment that is encouraging and empowering along with active participation in the decision-making process make caregivers gain control and boost their levels of hope. Crucially, nurses need to be mindful of their capacity in influencing hope sustainability within families.

Encouraging family carers to share their stories about challenges in their lives and exploring how these challenges demonstrate courage and optimism can enhance hope (Herth 2001). Hope is important in the adjustment process following trauma, disability or chronic illness, and the ability to maintain hope in the face of significant family disruption is both an affective and cognitive coping–response intervention. Understanding and acknowledging antecedents of hope, such as the major challenge of adopting the caregiving role, and all that it entails, such as loss and crisis, may help to stimulate hope.

Although the role of hope in helping individuals and their relatives has been explored over the years by nursing researchers, the challenge in supporting families and caregivers is to understand how to facilitate, foster and support hope. Further research is required that explores the interaction between hope-enhancing strategies and positive outcomes.

Key Points

- Nurses can play a pivotal role in fostering hope in family carers, which can also indirectly effect care recipients.
- Instilling hope starts with establishing a therapeutic relationship between the nurse and carer and is a subtle intangible process.
- Maintaining and fostering hope may help carers get though difficult situations, achieve meaning and achieve desired goals.
- Limited evidence exists to support strategies for fostering hope in family carers.

Fostering Resilience

To promote resilience in caregivers, it is necessary to have both internal and external resources available to provide structure and assist families in being able to cope (as discussed in Chapter 3). Skilled and resourceful nurses can access the level of stress in family carers through regular contact them and by providing space and time to discuss their fears and hope aspirations as well as daily challenges in caring. Nurses who adopt an empathetic approach when dealing with families and carers are able to then gauge their vulnerability and resilience. An increased understanding of the process involved in growing from adversity may enable nurses to better accomplish these facets of care and assist families and caregivers in their progression towards wellness, growth and development. Good partnership with the family is an essential aspect in providing care; hence, nurses should view the family as a positive influence and include them in their assessments and interventions. Families in turn can help the patient to comply and adhere with treatment and care management and help to increase patient resilience by providing support and management. In summary, family caregivers may be able to, with time, come to terms with the challenges that they face in their role with appropriate and timely support.

Key Points

- Carers need education and support to perform their caregiving role effectively.
- Support and interventions need to be individualised to the family carer.
- Education is a fundamental aspect of nursing care, and facilitating learning and empowering family caregivers are crucial in the pursuit of a meaningful and hopeful life.
- Continued research is necessary to help determine which interventions offer the best chance of improving the caregiving experience.
- By listening to families and carers, nurses can better understand and meet their psychosocial and spiritual needs.

Chapter Summary

Throughout this chapter, we have been aware that regardless of the intervention, the underpinning principles of nursing rely on good communication skills, empathy and compassion. Within the discussions on assessment, these principles can be interwoven and applied throughout each assessment and reassessment encounter. Of course, engaging with families and carers in positive and empathic ways can pose many challenges, for example, having adequate time and a calm environment. Arguably, such principles might seem idealistic but in fact as nurses adapting to circumstances and different contexts aligns to our professional strengths and one that we often thrive upon. Providing tailored interventions for the benefit of family caregivers cannot be undervalued or understated, as their reach can be enormous. Ways to offer support and information as discussed can vary but the overarching message is to offer support and information continually and to notably see support and information needs along a continuum. Having dialogues and securing a positive triad relationship between nurse, carer and care recipient are vital in regard to any intervention and encounter. As stated at the outset of this chapter, the ultimate goal is to promote salutogenesis through understanding and appropriate interventions. Finally, we are not suggesting that nurses are expected to deliver all the interventions outlined in this chapter but that they have a vital role in creating awareness of the plight of carers and families and should contribute towards good signposting in providing service to meet individual needs. In Chapter 7, we will focus on working *with* carers and families; in particular, we will look at lost opportunities for engagement with caregivers and where many of the interventions mentioned here could be repeated.

References

Agard AS and Lomborg K. (2010) Flexible family visitation in the intensive care unit: Nurses' decision-making. *Journal of Clinical Nursing* 20: 1106–1114.

Antonovsky A. (1979) *Health, Stress and Coping.* San Francisco, CA: Jossey-Bass.

Bambara JK, Owsley C, Wadley V, Martin R, Porter C and Dreer LE. (2009) Family caregiver social problem-solving abilities and adjustment to caring for a relative with vision loss. *Investigative Ophthalmology & Visual Science* 50(4): 1585–1592.

Berry JW, Elliott TR, Grant JS, Edwards G and Fine PR. (2012) Does problem-solving training for family caregivers benefit their care recipients with severe disabilities? A latent growth model of the project CLUES randomized clinical trial. *Rehabilitation Psychology* 57(2): 98–112.

Boss P. (1999) *Ambiguous Loss.* Cambridge, MA: Harvard University Press.

Boss P. (2004) Ambiguous loss research, theory, and practice: Reflections after 9/11. *Journal of Marriage and Family* 66(3): 551–566.

Boss P. (2006) *Loss Trauma and Resilience.* New York: W.W. Norton & Company.

Care Act. (2014) The Stationery Office, London, UK http://www.legislation.gov.uk/ukpga/2014/23/pdfs/ukpga_20140023_en.pdf (accessed 22 June 2015).

Carers UK. (2013) Supporting working carers: The benefits of families, business and the economy. Final report of the carers in employment task and finish group. London, UK: Carers UK.

Cattan M, White M, Bond J and Learmouth A. (2005) Preventing social isolation and loneliness among older people: A systematic review of health promotion interventions. *Ageing & Society* 25(1): 41–67.

Chung DS and Kim S. (2007) Characteristics of cancer blog users. *Journal of the Medical Library Association* 95(4): 445.

Cox C. (1997) Findings from a statewide program of respite care: A comparison of service users, stoppers, and nonusers. *The Gerontologist* 37: 511–517.

Damrosch SP and Perry LA. (1989) Self-reported adjustment, chronic sorrow, and coping of parents of children with down syndrome. *Nursing Research* 38: 25–30.

Dickens AP, Richards SH, Greaves CJ and Campbell JL. (2011) Interventions targeting social isolation in older people: A systematic review. [Research Support, Non-U.S. Gov't Review]. *BMC Public Health* 11: 647.

D'Zurilla T and Nezu A. (2007) *Problem Solving Therapy: A Positive Approach to Clinical Intervention*, 3rd ed. New York: Springer Publishing Company.

Elliott TR and Berry JW. (2009) Brief problem-solving training for family caregivers of persons with recent-onset spinal cord injury: A randomized controlled trial. *Journal of Clinical Psychology* 65: 406–422.

Elliott TR, Berry JW and Grant JS. (2009) Problem-solving training for family caregivers of women with disabilities: A randomized clinical trial. *Behaviour Research and Therapy* 47(7): 548–558.

Elliott TR, Brossart D, Berry JW and Fine PR. (2008) Problem-solving training via videoconferencing for family caregivers of persons with spinal cord injuries: A randomized controlled trial. *Behaviour Research and Therapy* 46: 1220–1229.

Farvaque N. (2013) Developing personal and household services in the EU. A focus on household activities. Report for the DG Employment, Social Affairs and Social Inclusion. Lille, France: Orseu.

Fowler NR, Hansen AS, Barnato AE and Garand L. (2013) Association between anticipatory grief and problem solving among family caregivers of persons with cognitive impairment. *Journal of Aging and Health* 25(3): 493–509.

Gaugler JE, Jarrott SE, Zarit SH, Stephens MP, Townsend A and Greene R. (2003) Respite for dementia caregivers: The effects of adult day service use on caregiving hours and care demands. *International Psychogeriatrics* 15: 37–58.

Given BA, Given CW and Sherwood PR. (2012) Family and caregiver needs over the course of the cancer trajectory. *Journal of Supportive Oncology* 10(2): 57–64.

Grant JS, Elliott TR, Weaver M, Bartolucci AA and Giger JN. (2002) Telephone intervention with family caregivers of stroke survivors after rehabilitation. *Stroke* 33(8): 2060–2065.

Herth KA. (2001) Development and implementation of a hope intervention program. *Oncology Nursing Forum* 28: 1009–1017.

Jacelon C and Imperio K. (2005) Participant diaries as a source of data in research with older adults. *Qualitative Health Research* 15: 991–997.

Johansson AK and Grimby A. (2011) Anticipatory grief among close relatives of patients in hospice and palliative wards. *American Journal of Hospice & Palliative Medicine* 29(2): 134–138.

Knapp M, Bauer A, Perkins M and Snell T. (2010) Building community capacity: Making an economic case. PSSRU discussion paper 2772. London, UK: PSSRU. http://eprints.lse. ac.uk/33163/1/dp2772.pdf (accessed 29 June 2015).

Kosloski K and Montgomery R. (1995) The impact of respite use on nursing home placement. *The Gerontologist* 35: 67–74.

Lauder W, Mummery K and Sharkey S. (2006) Social capital, age and religiosity in people who are lonely. *Journal of Clinical Nursing* 15(3): 334–340.

Lui MH, Ross FM and Thompson DR. (2005) Supporting family caregivers in stroke care: A review of the evidence for problem solving. *Stroke* 36(11): 2514–2522.

Lazarus RS and Folkman S. (1984) *Stress Appraisal and Coping.* New York: Springer.

Marmot M. (2010) *Fair Society, Healthy Lives: The Marmot Review.* London, UK: The Marmot Review.

Marwit SJ and Meuser TM. (2005) Development of a short form inventory to assess grief in caregivers of dementia patients. *Death Studies* 29: 191–205.

Masi CM, Chen HY, Hawkley LC and Cacioppo JT. (2011) A meta-analysis of interventions to reduce loneliness. [Meta-Analysis Research Support, N.I.H., Extramural Research Support, Non-U.S. Gov't Review]. *Personality and Social Psychology Review* 15(3): 219–266.

Mead N, Lester H, Chew-Graham C, Gask L and Bower P. (2010) Effects of befriending on depressive symptoms and distress: Systematic review and meta-analysis. *British Journal of Psychiatry* 196(2): 96–101.

Mentoring and Befriending Foundation (MBF). (2010) Befriending works: Building resilience in local communities. Manchester, UK: MBF

Miller JF. (1991) Developing and maintaining hope in families of the critically ill. *AACN Clinical Issues in Critical Care Nursing* 2: 307–365.

Papacharissi Z. (2004) Democracy online: Civility, politeness, and the democratic potential of online discussion groups. *New Media & Society* 6: 259–283.

Pennebaker JW. (1997) Writing about emotional experiences as a therapeutic process. *Psychological Science* 8(3): 162–166.

Pennebaker JW. (1999) Forming a story: The health benefits of narrative. *Journal of Clinical Psychology* 55(10): 1243–1254.

Phillipson L, Magee C and Jones SC. (2013) Why carers of people with dementia do not utilise out-of-home respite services. *Health and Social Care in the Community* 21(4): 411–422.

Plowfield LA. (1999) Living a nightmare: Family experiences of waiting following neurological crisis. *Journal of Neuroscience Nursing* 31(4): 231–238.

Quinn C, Clare L, McGuiness T and Woods RT. (2012) The impact of relationships, motivation and meanings on dementia caregivers outcomes. *International Psychogeriatrics* 24: 1816–1826.

Quinn C, Clare L and Woods RT. (2010) The impact of motivations and meanings on the wellbeing of caregivers of people with dementia: A systematic review *International Psychogeriatrics* 22(1): 43–55.

Rando TA. (2000) *Clinical Dimensions of Anticipatory Mourning: Theory Practice in Working with the Dying, Their Loved Ones and Their Caregivers.* Champaign, IL: Lexington Books.

Rivera P, Elliott TR, Berry J and Grant J. (2008) Problem-solving training for family caregivers of persons with traumatic brain injuries: A randomized controlled trial. *Archives of Physical Medicine and Rehabilitation* 89: 931–941.

Scherbring M. (2002). Effect of caregiver perception of preparedness on burden in an oncology population. *Oncology Nursing Forum* 29(6): E70–E76.

Snyder CR. (1994) *The Psychology of Hope: You can Get There from Here.* New York: Free Press.

Snyder CR. (2000) The past and possible futures of hope. *Journal of Social and Clinical Psychology* 19: 11–28.

Stirling CM, Dwan CA and McKenzie AR. (2014) Why carers use adult day respite: A mixed method case study. *BMC Health Services Research* 14: 245.

Turner D and Stokes L. (2006) Hope promoting strategies of registered nurses. *Journal of Advanced Nursing* 56: 363–372.

United Nations. (2013) Ageing populations. http://www.un.org/en/development/desa/population/publications/dataset/urban/profilesOfAgeing2013.shtml (accessed 29 June 2015).

Ure C. (2015) What is breast cancer 'survivorship'? A discursive psychological analysis of a blogger's lived experiences of the media's representation of being a breast cancers survivor. *Psychology of Women Section Review* 17: 41–47. https://www.academia.edu/12070143/Psychology_of_Women_Section_Review_Issue_17 (accessed 1.7.15).

Verhaeghe S, van Zuuren FF, Defloor T, Dujnstee MSH and Grypdonck MHF. (2007a) The process and meaning of hope for family members of traumatic coma patients in intensive care. *Qualitative Health Research* 17: 730–743.

Verhaeghe ST, van Zuuren FJ, Defloor T, Duijnstee MS and Grypdonck MH. (2007b) How does information influence hope in family members of traumatic coma patients in intensive care unit? *Journal of Clinical Nursing* 16(8): 1488–1497.

Wade SL, Carey J and Wolfe CR. (2006) An online family intervention to reduce parental distress following pediatric brain injury. *Journal of Consulting and Clinical Psychology* 74: 445–454.

WHO. (2014) http://www.who.int/ageing/about/facts/en/ (accessed 25 June 2015).

Windle K, Francis F and Coomber C. (2011) Preventing loneliness and social isolation: Interventions and outcomes. Research Briefing 39. London, UK: Social Care Institute for Excellence. http://www.scie.org.uk/publications/briefings/files/briefing39.pdf (accessed 29 June 2015).

Useful Links

Admiral nurses are specialist dementia nurses in the United Kingdom who give much-needed practical and emotional support to family carers, as well as to persons with dementia: http://www.dementiauk.org/what-we-do/admiral-nurses.

Care and Respite Support Services is a charity that supports carers to help them make a life outside caring in the North West of England: http://www.careandrespitesupportservices.co.uk/.

Dementia Carer is a resource for carers of people with dementia: http://www.dementiacarer.net/.

Marie Curie Care and Support offers expert care, guidance and support for people living with any terminal illness and for their families in the United Kingdom: https://www.mariecurie.org.uk.

Mentoring and befriending network is a free network for anyone interested in the growth and development of mentoring and befriending. Available resources include help setting up or developing a mentoring or befriending service and practical support for volunteering: http://www.mandbf.org.

Social Inclusion and Loneliness research hub – provides links to academic research units, charities and funders which focus on topics such as social inclusion and loneliness in ageing: http://www.ageuk.org.uk/professional-resources-home/knowledge-hub-evidence-statistics/research-community/social-inclusion-and-loneliness-research/.

Start Training Academy is aimed at improving the skills of carers for people with dementia by offering online training modules in dementia all over Europe: http://startraining.eu/index.php/en/.

SupportLine offers confidential emotional support for children, young adults and adults, especially for people who feel socially isolated: http://www.supportline.org.uk/.

The Campaign to End Loneliness is a campaign which draws on research and inspiration from across the United Kingdom to offer ideas to both individuals and those working with older people: www.campaigntoendloneliness.org.uk/.

The QNI was originally established in 1887 to train district nurses to treat patients in their own homes. Today their remit is wider, but their core aim remains the same: 'we want high-quality nursing care to be available to people in the community and in their own homes': http://www.qni.org.uk/for_nurses.

The Technology Enabled Care Services (TECS) Resource: http://www.england.nhs.uk/ourwork/qual-clin-lead/tecs/.

Young Carers is a carers trust: www.youngcarers.net.

Twitter Accounts
@Carers

7

Working with Families and Carers

Looking back, a simple 'how are you?' would have helped and if I could say anything it would be to ask, be empathetic and notice us.

Sophie (Young carer)

Introduction

It is in this final chapter that we discuss more of the practical aspects of working *with* families and carers. Having explored interventions in some detail in Chapter 6, notably for supporting families and carers, we now wish to shift the emphasis towards opportunities, and, by association, obstacles that can hinder working with families and carers. By now you will have gathered that we believe strongly in an inclusive and participatory approach to working with families and carers in all care settings. Yet we would be naïve to suggest or imply that such an endeavour and desire is easy; far from it, challenges are everywhere. In fact, we acknowledge that you could have lots of positive experiences. You may also partake in excellent practice by overcoming obstacles and adopting an integrated all-inclusive and effective working dynamic relationship which encompasses every aspect of engagement with families and carers. Throughout this book, we have highlighted how research has shown the importance of involving families and carers in caring for and in the treatment of their loved ones. As outlined in Chapter 2, both family-centred care (FCC) and family-centred practice rest upon seeing the family and patient as a single unit of care in the context that together they should participate in decisions about their own care (Galvin et al. 2000). We know that increased participation and collaboration result in improved patient outcomes such as increased satisfaction with care, increased feelings of control over health, increased feelings of well-being and better compliance with prescribed treatments (Dalton 2003). It is also well established that collaborative approaches to care enhance quality and safety of care along with increased coordination and efficiency of care. Importantly because nurses spend a lot of time with patients, they affect both the patient experiences of care and their families.

Collaborative opportunities with family caregivers as partners in care add to such positive outcomes. However, our experience and research portray a landscape that is in need of improvements and that in busy healthcare settings opportunities can be lost. The evidence base is clear that families and carers for the most part contribute significantly to the lives of the sick, ill and disabled (Levine 2004); society would indeed be a worse place if they didn't. As such, it is imperative that we ensure to protect everyone in our midst with dignity and personhood and that no one is 'dehumanised' or discounted in any care setting. This chapter in its entirety seeks to inspire, motivate and energise you to 'look for signs' and thus opportunities where you can engage *with* families and carers.

In seeking to emphasise some of the salient points presented in this chapter, we have invited a number carers to share examples from their story by way of highlights. To set the scene, we start with a pertinent and powerful comment from an adult support care manager based at a Carers Centre. You will note a couple of fundamental key questions that you ought to be asking consistently in planning transfer of care to the home.

Working with Families and Carers – Some Thoughts from Helen...

Amongst nursing staff the will to identify and support carers exists; however, in the 'busyness' of healthcare settings, be it hospitals, clinics, GP surgeries or home visits, the opportunities to refer or signpost carers and families to local Carers Centre support services is often lost or missed.

Identifying families and carers is part of the culture throughout services, from frontline admin staff to clinicians and healthcare professionals, to ensure that carers will get the information and support they need and deserve. Carers may not need support immediately, but knowing where they can turn, before they reach a crisis point, could prevent future readmissions, deterioration in carer's health or potential problems in their caring roles.

By asking the questions 'do you look after someone?' or 'does someone look after you?' especially around discharge planning, has the potential to identify carers, young adult carers or young carers, but making that next step to refer carers to a local Carers Centre is crucial. The process to refer carers to these centres needs to be simple and direct – by phone calls or referral forms on a website.

The importance in this example for nursing is carer awareness and being mindful of asking about who looks after whom and knowing where to signpost people to. We are not suggesting that nurses are totally responsible for support; far from it, it is a collective endeavour. However, opportunities exist in their simplest form and can be exploited for the holistic benefit of families and their carers.

Brief Policy Context

Real people and real stories are hugely powerful and meaningful. Hearing and listening to the voices of caregivers and close family has gathered momentum over the past 5 years or so in the NHS. For example, valuing carers was made most explicit in the UK government's carers' strategy (England) in 2008 and is to be achieved by 2018, where the overarching objective 'that carers are recognised and supported as an expert care partners' (UK Government 2008) was stated. In support, a notable turning point in reinforcing valuing patients and their families evolved in the United Kingdom as a consequence of the Francis Inquiry Report in 2013 (Francis Report 2013), according to which leadership, culture and respect for patients and their families were flagged as being core attributes in any care setting. A key message that was reinforced in the United Kingdom was the principle of putting the patient at the heart of everything, i.e., 'patients' needs come first and the values of patient-centred care' (The Kings Fund 2013, p. 7). On the one hand, public harm as a result of failure in caregiving at the Mid Staffordshire NHS Foundation Trust in England (Francis 2013) sent shockwaves across the United Kingdom and throughout the NHS and thus public confidence was affected and a period of uncertainty prevailed. Yet at the same time, emphasis was placed upon what the public can expect and indeed deserve in terms of compassionate care, in particular, for those who are most at risk and vulnerable. Rethinking public trust became a national priority and numerous policy reactions arose such as 'Compassion in Practice' that set out the '6 Cs'* (DH 2012).

At the same time, in 2013, the NHS friends and family test (FFT) was introduced (DH 2013) to provide an opportunity to ask patients whether they would recommend hospital wards, A&E departments and maternity services to their friends and family if they needed similar care or treatment (DH 2013). FFT is recognised as a quick feedback method on the quality of care given, so that hospitals can have a better understanding of the needs of their patients so as to assist in improvements. Arguably, obtaining a snapshot view that does not wholly capture 'experience', and as the FFT is structured around a few standard questions derived from a Net Promoter management tool from the private sector to gauge customer loyalty, and is not without critiques. Conversely, obtaining feedback from, and engaging with, family caregivers in different contexts and over time is an activity being undertaken by many healthcare providers using innovative methods. However, the voice and considerations of service users and their caregivers are captured; the prime underpinning ethos is one that should be informed by the values, ethics and moral beliefs of human caring and kindness. Dewar and Christley (2013), in their critical analysis of the policy drive for 'compassion in practice' (DH 2012), draw attention to the tensions of simplifying compassionate practice into 6 Cs and the need for much more involvement of families, patients and staff in seeking to transform a values-based culture. In our experience of working *with* families and carers, a triad partnership comprising the patient, nurse and caregiver (family) strengthens relationships and experiences for all concerned. This may be a familiar concept, and yet many authors allude to the notion of triad partnerships, for example, Dalton's (2013) theory of *collaborative decision-making in nursing practice for a triad*, which seeks to build upon decision making theories. Dalton's research highlights the benefits of caregiver's inclusion in advancing the 'client–caregiver–nurse relationship'. Interestingly, the Triangle of Care was incorporated into guidance launched in 2010 jointly between Carers Trust and the National Mental Health Development Unit (Carers Trust 2010). Here, the emphasis is on better local strategic involvement of carers and families in the care planning and treatment of people with mental illness. The concept of a triangle, see Figure 7.1, was proposed through collaboration with many carers as 'a therapeutic alliance between service user, staff and carer that promotes safety, supports recovery and sustains well-being' (Carers Trust 2010, p. 6).

Thinking Box

Are you familiar with notions of triangle of care or triad theory?

How do you feel about it?

How does it work for you?

On recalling Chapter 1 and Benner et al. (1999), do you think this triangle or triad connects with the phenomenon of the 'human pull' and helps carers and nurses to come together with their different 'reaching out' factors and incentives?

We have chosen to highlight this background context by reiterating the evidence that cannot be disputed: that carers are a growing population in all societies and that their inclusion is vital in every aspect of care planning and decision-making – as genuine partners.

---

* This policy introduces six fundamental values: care, compassion, competence, communication, courage and commitment (commonly referred to as the 6 Cs).

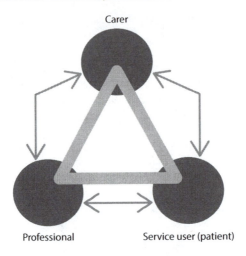

Figure 7.1 Carers trust: Triangle of Care. (Adapted from Carers Trust, *The Triangle of Care: Carers Included: A Guide to Best Practice in Acute Mental Health Care*, Carers Trust, London, UK., 2010, p. 6, http://www.rcn.org.uk/_data/assets/pdf_file/0009/549063/Triangle_of_Care_-_Carers_Included_Sept_2013.pdf, accessed 17 July 2015.)

The following account from a patient highlights insights into the appreciation and meanings of the actions of a nurse who is compassionate in using *human pull* by being kind and caring towards both Rob and his wife – the family carer. Perhaps jot down some notes on how this story makes you feel and what you can learn from it.

Story 1 – From Rob

My last bout of surgery was in October 2013, and it went well, and after a couple of days of adjusting to new drugs, I was sent home where I developed a rather disturbing side effect of the surgery. While I'd been made aware of this potential side effect prior to surgery, it remained disturbing and my wife was at a loss as to what to do to help. My whole body had a permanent sensation of pins and needles especially my head where my brain felt as though it was electrically charged. I contacted my renal unit and was asked to attend clinic for more blood tests.... My wife accompanied me to the renal unit the following morning by which time I was in some distress and my ashen-faced wife was extremely concerned for my welfare, not really understanding what was happening to me. The results of the blood tests would take a few hours to arrive so we decided to go and get a drink at the hospital café. On the way there I recognised one of the specialist transplant nurses that I hadn't seen for some time and said "Hello" in passing. She returned the greeting but she could tell that all was not well and came over and gave both of us a huge hug. We explained the situation and she took us to one side, all the while gently holding my wife's hand, assured us that the problem was a relatively common side effect and that all would be well in a day or two. Throughout our brief discussion her eyes rarely left my wife, instinctively understanding that while I'd be receiving great care my wife would still have that overwhelming worry and sense of helplessness. Feeling less anxious we parted, had our drink and awaited the results of the blood tests. In the end, my tests resulted in an amended prescription. So, we left the unit and saw the same nurse walking toward us down the main corridor, this time my wife hugged her, as she'd found time to address my concerns while focusing on my wife's well-being above everything else in her working day.

This act of kindness and thoughtfulness, as a therapeutic 'intervention', undertaken by the nurse has remained a constant positive and meaningful experience for Rob and his wife. Arguably, this is opportunistic in nature on the part of the nurse, who seemingly 'reached out' and offered support and by doing so contributed towards reducing anxiety and emotional turmoil for both caregiver and patient. We believe that for the most part nurses are committed to acts of kindness and empathy, and such an impact has long-lasting effects on carers and families. However, lost opportunities arise, and as Sophie articulated at the very outset of this chapter, 'notice us', a simple acknowledgement can be massive and symbolic of a caring and kind culture.

Context of Hospitalisation

Within the context of being in hospital numerous opportunities arise to get information about family caring and the impact of illness and care from the perspectives of family caregivers. In other words, finding ways to draw upon family caregivers experiences so as to help their loved one is essential. Lowson et al. (2013) suggest that further attention should be paid to the expertise, contribution and support of family carers within institutional settings, as well as care provided at home. At this juncture, we thought it would be worthwhile to think about, in the context of hospitalisation, how to interact and engage with visitors during visiting times. Interaction with visitors and relatives is a challenging task and arguably requires complex skills. A balancing act is often required between the needs of the patient, relatives and staff (Bube 2002). As nurse educators, we often ask student nurses *what do you do during visiting hours* and the responses are insightful, from minimal contact to some engagement to stating 'no contact'. Maybe at this point you would like to think about what you do [make some notes]. It is in this context that opportunities exist to identify family caregivers and engage with them as partners in care. Forming a relationship through face-to-face communication with both patients and their relatives is a core competence of nursing (Solli et al. 2015). Nurses are ideally placed as close carers of patients to support and provide information to caregivers but more than that to seek to understand the role of caregivers and their tasks. Thus, opportunities are plenty during hospitalisation to discuss caring skills and to obtain knowledge and understanding of treatments; probably visiting times offer a 'window of opportunity' for this to happen.

Of course practices during visiting times and experiences will vary and highly depend upon the environment, culture and leadership. Visitation strategies differ considerably in the United Kingdom and traditions play a huge role rather than an evidence base per se. That said, in the United Kingdom we see contemporary visitation practices and philosophies shifting towards flexible visitation in that relatives can visit at any time so long as it does not interfere with the patient's dignity, safety and privacy. We will now draw our attention to visitation in some detail.

Visitation

Interestingly, hospitals are places of work for healthcare professionals and other staff, but for many visitors and relatives, hospitals can feel strange and intimidating. The meanings and constructions that people attach to hospitals inform their behaviours and activities to some extent. Place of care matters, and care environments, by their nature of being an institution, have 'rules' and thus impact those working and residing in shared places, e.g., hospital wards

(Wray 2012). We know that tensions can exist between wards being a workspace for staff whereby they are in control of the environment (Nash 2002) alongside being a place of rest and recuperation. Interestingly, the atmosphere of a ward in terms of the *feel of the place* (Wray 2011) alongside visitation arrangements influences how visitors feel about the place of care and their perceptions of nursing values and quality of care. Place and space matter as both impact the sense of wellness, interpretations of caregiving and meanings people attach to care settings. Clarifying our values about the contribution and involvement of patients' relatives can go some way to informing visitation practices. In the following short story, a family caregiver mentions the inflexibility that can happen, but more importantly the potential impact of communication breakdown and the subsequent attitude.

Story 2 – Family Carer

I lived some distance away from my mum and being in fulltime work had limited possibilities to visit her in hospital during the set times, so I would text her (she is quite a techno mum for her age) and she would be happy with that. But I wanted to see her in person especially after her surgery (I would be her main carer when she went home), so I rang the ward to ask if this would be okay, they were not keen but I seemed to persuade them that I could go out of the set hours. On this basis, I drove over to the hospital (took an hour) and when I got there the ward door was locked. I rang the bell and after what felt like ages a nurse came and said 'oh you're not allowed at this time'. I pleaded and said I had rung up previously to ask, the nurse rolled her eyes and said wait there. After 10 minutes, another nurse came and said reluctantly 'okay you can come in but only for 10 minutes'. I felt awful to have bothered them, in fact it felt like I was a nuisance and I worried it might affect my mum. I would not complain and they were good to mum, but at times like this, a better attitude would have helped and to have passed on the information.

Thinking Box

Does this story sound familiar?

How might you have dealt with this?

What informs/drives your visitation practices? Are these evidence based?

In debates about visitation (and they are plentiful) in 2011, the RCN made a statement to the BBC suggesting that hospital visiting times should be extended, so patients' relatives can become more involved in their care. The then head of the Royal College of Nursing, Peter Carter, said, '... [we] do not want relatives performing tasks nurses were employed to carry out, but that there were "real benefits" for patients when family members helped with care' (BBC 2011). As part of a Florence Nightingale Foundation Travel Scholarship, Wray undertook a study in 2015 to look at family and carer involvement in Denmark and Spain and found visiting arrangements differed. For example, in Denmark, close family are encouraged to visit the very sick and ill patients, and family wings exist in hospitals to support access. However, more distant family, young children or acquaintances are discouraged from visiting hospitals (although a criterion exists for this to happen). In Spain, a primary carer is identified on admission and for the most part takes a lead role in supporting the patient and staff; consideration to the benefits of distant family, young children or acquaintances is explored by nurses in consultation with patients. We are not suggesting that visitation strategies need to be changed or that 'one size fits all', but there is room to reflect as to the purpose and benefits of visiting arrangements. The examples highlighted from Denmark and Spain are closely associated with minimal hospital-acquired infection rates, cultural beliefs and a drive towards reducing or preventing hospital stays. Day surgery and day care are massive alternatives in Denmark, for example. It is in learning about others that we can explore opportunities for improving our own visitation strategies, as even at a micro level, differences are experienced by families and carers. You can perhaps think of some of these differences, but then how do we explain them to people? We have no absolute solutions but suggest one of the most important factors: engagement with carers during visiting times is not overlooked. Moving on to consider other involvement opportunities, we now turn to specific assessments such as the ABCDE framework (Resuscitation Council UK 2000).

ABCDEF Assessment

It is important to involve relatives (caregivers) during admission in care settings, such as ICU and rehabilitation (Agard and Maindl 2009), as they are valuable sources of information and can enable more personalised care for the patient. In particular, opportunities exist in assessing patients at risk of rapid deterioration with the well-established and commonly used ABCDE framework (Resuscitation Council UK 2000; Allen 2004). A crucial element of this assessment is obtaining information from family or friends who could add further evidence regarding the circumstance. In our view, this is a crucial missed opportunity – the F dimension (see Figure 7.2). Of course in some situations F may not apply, but it is a useful addition to consider. For example, within neuroscience care, such as the onset of a stroke or seizure, accurate patient history is critical to assessment and treatment processes, and thus it is recommended to involve the family or friend (carer) whose insights can add vital information to the assessment process.

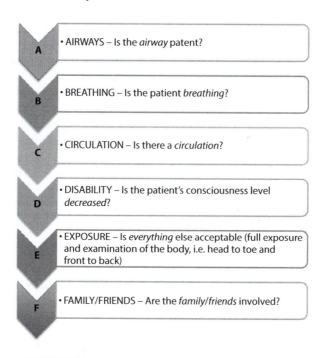

A • AIRWAYS – Is the *airway* patent?

B • BREATHING – Is the patient *breathing*?

C • CIRCULATION – Is there a *circulation*?

D • DISABILITY – Is the patient's consciousness level *decreased*?

E • EXPOSURE – Is *everything* else acceptable (full exposure and examination of the body, i.e. head to toe and front to back)

F • FAMILY/FRIENDS – Are the *family/friends* involved?

Figure 7.2 Adapted ABCDE (F) framework to include family/friends.

Protected Meal Times

Increased rate of malnutrition amongst adult patients as a result of longer hospital stays (NPSA 2006) was the key driver in improving mealtime experiences through 'protected mealtimes (PM)'. For some patients, especially older patients, nutritional status could already have been compromised and once in hospital are at risk of deteriorating further (Stratton et al. 2003). As a measure to respond to the mealtime environment, interruptions and patient's experience and to enhance nutrient intake, a UK-wide initiative of protected mealtimes was established (NPSA 2006; DH 2007). Hailed as the absolute way forward for improving nutritional care and intake, this initiative has unfortunately had varied effects. For example, Hickson et al. (2011), in their observational study in a large teaching hospital, found only minor improvements in mealtime experiences following the implementation of PM and that the expected macronutrient intake did not improve. Within the context of busy wards, tension can arise in securing time and accountability to encouraging patients to eat well and improve their nutritional intake in a consistent manner. Once again, there are numerous benefits and opportunities for a family caregiver to help and play a key role in feeding patients and improving mealtime experience. The nature of this involvement aligns to FCC whereby families are integral to care delivery and care encounters (Turnbull and Turnbull 2001). Perhaps a philosophical underpinning has been overlooked in how PM has been implemented in that the mealtime experience is more than just obtaining 'nutrients'. Eating is also a social and personal encounter, and thus being ill compounds one's desires to eat. Clearly, there is scope and potential for family carers to play a vital role in PM. However, careful considerations of the logistics need to be made, but undeniably benefits of PM for patients do exist. Research in this area is rather sparse and equivocal in terms of the individual and social aspect of eating in hospital. As discussed in Chapter 1, caregivers undertake different roles and perform differing tasks (direct and indirect); and the inclusion of their knowledge base and experience could be hugely advantageous in seeking to improve nutritional intake. Conversely, revelations may well unfold in regard of a caregiver's knowledge of food/nutrients (or lack of) and as such learning and educational opportunities could unfold. Arguably, involvement as a consequence of participation in mealtimes complements the values of collaboration and partnerships, whereby goals between patients, family caregivers and professionals can be mutually agreed (Walker and Dewar 2001; Dalton 2003).

Discharge Planning

There is no doubt that globally shorter stays in hospital have become the norm within contemporary healthcare irrespective of the health breakdown and reason for being in hospital. Consequently, the shift in focus from the acute care sector to the home is supported more by community care services and has implications for family caregivers. Discharge or care transfer is an essential part of care management in any setting (DH 2010), and therefore early discharge means that a major part of recovery will be taking place within the home and community (DH 2003). However, the transition from hospital to home is well recognised as a cause of great uncertainty and stress. This could be attributed to two key factors – first is the realisation of the consequences of the illness or condition and what might be involved, and second is the shift in responsibility back to the family from healthcare professionals. At the same time, families can often experience tremendous pressure due to major changes in their lives (as well as the patients) caused by critical illness and health breakdown of their loved ones. Additional caregiving roles may well unfold and be expected of the family or indeed caregiving as a loved one's disease or illness is realised, and many aspects of this role maybe unfamiliar to them. In either case, the nature of caring and expertise to carry out the tasks can be complex and create anxiety for the family caregiver as we have seen in Chapter 5. Yet as 'secondary patients', carers can often feel unprepared to provide care, have limited knowledge in regard to performing adequate care and have received little guidance or training from healthcare professionals (Reinhard et al. 2008). And yet it is well known within the literature that supporting carers during the process of discharge can avoid delayed discharges, reduce re-admissions, improve recovery of the care recipient and enable care to continue (Borthwick et al. 2009; Stone 2014). Carer preparedness is therefore crucial if they are expected to continue to provide 'good and proper' care. Seeking opportunities to interact with family caregivers about after-care needs ought to commence as an integral part of admission and on-going assessments. The following story from a family caregiver offers some insights into seeing beyond immediate circumstances.

Story 3 – Mrs C

Mrs C, who is 92 and is the main carer for her husband, who she says is forgetful*, is admitted to a busy ward with dehydration following an episode of food poisoning in order for her kidney function to be monitored, rehydration and if needed rehabilitation. Prior to admission, they were both living independently with minimal support from her daughter. Mrs C made a slow but good recovery and started eating and drinking independently and according to ward staff, became self-caring, although her daughter noticed her cognition was impaired when compared to pre-admission. Mr C had noticeably deteriorated without his wife's support and had started to wander outside the home at night and become disoriented to time and place. Discharge was arranged for Mrs C with relatives being asked if they could arrange transport the following day. Mrs C's daughter asked if support had been arranged because they had not been involved in the discharge planning process and were assured 'everything was in place for discharge'.

What transpired was that Mrs C was discharged and was taken home by her daughter. The take-home medication was not available at the time but her daughter was reassured that this could be collected later that day. According to her discharge care plan, no support package had been arranged for Mrs C who was now unable to remember where things were in her home and struggled to remember how to make a drink or snack. Mr C continued to wander and was kindly brought home by people in the village where they lived from varying distances from their home. On contacting the ward to check what, if any, support was planned, she was told 'No' and that her mother had reassured staff that she 'was fine'. Things at home quickly reached a crisis point after day one of discharge, Mrs C was unable to self-medicate, cook or care for

---

* Diagnosed with dementia.

Mr C and emergency social care was arranged that gave both Mr and Mrs C support for a period of 6 weeks following her hospital admission. Gradually, over the next few weeks, Mrs C's condition improved and she managed at home with a continuing care package and much increased support from her family.

In reading this story, we suggest that you think about a few questions:

- How might you see beyond the immediate circumstances of Mrs C?
- How would you explore statements of 'being fine' in view of her age?
- At what point would you have involved at relative in planning discharge?

A key message here is that it is essential that relatives and carers are included in conversations when planning care to establish levels of self-care prior to and after illness or other crisis. As we have said from the outset, in busy healthcare settings, opportunities may be lost and so it is essential that structured conversations take place with vulnerable people, that the cared for and carers views are sought and acknowledged and that understanding is checked and established.

A dimension of the 'ebb and flow' of patients who are readmitted into hospital and the care responsibility shifts back to the hospital is that caregivers tend to 'watch over' the care (Agard et al. 2015). On the one hand, they are faced with handing back control and power to professionals as they grapple with their shifting role and the division of labour between themselves and nurses. But at the same time they seek to remain involved in decision-making processes. However, often their knowledge and expertise are not recognised or acknowledged by healthcare professionals (Lowson et al. 2013). We believe that nurses can profoundly change the typical pattern of events between caregivers and care recipients through enacting more empowering partnership approaches such as Dalton's (2003) theory of decision-making in nursing practice triads. By increasing interactions and collaborating *with* caregivers, nurses can influence feelings of control, sense of well-being, confidence and compliance with treatments. Sentiment and policy materials clearly exist (e.g. DH 2003, 2010; UK Government 2008) to facilitate smooth, inclusive and thoughtful planning to transfer care over to caregivers (discharge planning). Indeed, there is a strong health policy movement towards co-production and shared decision-making which rests upon collaboration, inclusive nature of 'others' and changing relationships between professionals, patients and carers. So more than ever it is imperative that an inclusive process within the realms of discharge planning happen as patients and caregivers benefit hugely in the short term and, more importantly, beyond.

Finding out about caregivers' health literacy is also a key aspect of ongoing assessment but certainly in relation to plans for going home. Where limited health literacy exists, finding ways to help family carers is important, especially for treatments involving medicines. We cannot assume that information given is understood, as people process information in different ways and as nurses we need to check their understanding. Slatyer et al. (2013) found in their study of older people readmitted to hospital that discharge readiness is an important aspect together with providing information so as to ensure carers and family understand and are prepared for future health crises. Given illness and disease trajectories alongside the ethos of self-care, we need to appreciate that the nature of support and information needs to change over time. We need to create proactive attitudes and facilitative communication strategies towards optimum discharge planning. As suggested by Helen (carers support manager; Working with Families and Carers box), questions such as 'do you look after someone?' or 'does someone look after you?' should be asked.

In light of the ongoing growth in day surgery, it is important to clarify to whom the care responsibility is being transferred and to ensure carers are well informed and prepared to take on this responsibility. Typically in day surgery, the responsibility of care is transferred to the patient and their relatives. Often, the person responsible is a partner or carer who may need to take leave from work and provide help with the activities of day living or direct tasks, recovery monitoring and providing emotional support, and this will vary according to the nature of surgery. Thus, opportunities need to be found to involve and engage carers in the whole process of discharging the patient to home. Interestingly in a study of discharge following day surgery, Mottram (2011) warns that assumptions about rapid recovery and self-care due to the nature of day surgery (which is becoming more complex and not just about minor operations) should not be made. Far from it, time should be dedicated in promoting self-care at home as Anne Mottram found that issues concerning unexpected occurrences following discharge caused lack of confidence in both patients and their carers on their ability to care for themselves or their loved ones (p. 3147). She also found a distinct lack of after-care in the community and lack of perceived support from primary care teams.

For the most part, we all have a responsibility to stop and think about the potential and real long-term gains from good discharge planning, such as reduced inappropriate readmissions (Slatyer et al. 2013), compliance with care and treatments and more satisfied caregivers and patients (Bradby 2014). By practising in this context, we are likely to be promoting salutogenesis, and as we have previously discussed, achieving well-being at this level should be our goal as nurses. In fact, The Queen's Nursing Institute has created an interactive learning resource for nurses with the objective to help community nurses to recognise and plan for the needs of carers and to signpost them to sources of support from voluntary organisations and other agencies (Bradby 2014; see http://www.qni.org.uk/ supporting_carers). We suggest that you take a look at this resource if you have not already; the information is accessible and very useful.

Relationships between Nurses and Caregivers

Irrespective of care setting, working *with* families and carers is enhanced by adopting genuine partnerships; for example, as mentioned in Chapters 1 and 2, the FCC approach results in improved family and patient satisfaction, reduced anxiety for the family and improved patient safety. However, clinical care settings are areas of complexity and being able to draw boundaries between accessing information about the family that enables facilitation of family goals and the family's rights and needs to privacy is a challenging one (Keen and Knox 2004). How might we seek to deal with this concern? On the one hand, if we are seeking to build mutual respect and trust in our encounters with families and carers, then forming close or distant relationships with them is necessary, which is reliant upon good communication skills. Concerns about maintaining confidentiality and patient privacy often emerge as tensions and issues in sharing across the 'triad' or triangle of care. But when we look at the research related to families, findings indicate that concerns regarding patient privacy are more of a problem for nurses than for patients and family members (Tobiano et al. 2012). Thus, care should be well thought through, not based on assumptions but through appropriate and open dialogue with the patient and caregivers. In some instances, it is possible to know the primary caregiver and have a good rapport and understanding. This is not always the case. However, it is important to remember that some carers may also be children and young people, and as such can be hidden or invisible.

In seeking to understand working *with* hidden and tertiary carers, and the opportunity for FCC in the context of dementia, we offer a commentary extract from some emerging research findings (see Box 7.1). We have chosen an extract that needs attention in

---

Box 7.1 Commentary extract: Lauren*, 12 years old, granddaughter of a woman with young-onset dementia

Lauren has been interviewed three times over a year about how her grandmother's young-onset dementia has affected her and her family. She is not her grandmother's 'carer'; her grandfather assumes the main responsibility of assisting her grandmother with the activities of daily living. Nevertheless, Lauren is clearly emotionally affected by tension within family relationships caused by her grandmother's condition, as the following quote demonstrates:

> sometimes she's happier, because she's trying to make the most out of what memory she's got left, but sometimes she's really batty and shouty and snaps at you for nothing, but then I get upset when she shouts at me, but then my granddad comes and speaks to her, and then my nana and granddad fall out because my nana's made me upset

When a serious and progressive illness occurs within a family context, it cannot be assumed that family members communicate with each other either about the nature of the condition or their response to it; for example, Lauren states:

> I didn't know it was a terminal disease... my granddad knew, my nana knew, and I went 'what, terminal? That means you're gonna die?' and they was like 'yeah did you not know that?' 'Cos they thought I knew but I didn't so that shocked me

Lauren remarks that the wider family rarely communicate about her grandmother's dementia and describes her own reasons for her reluctance to discuss the condition with them:

> I hate speaking to my mum about things, so my friends at school are the only people I would... because I'd never talk to my nana about it 'cos she'd probably get upset, and my granddad would, so I just speak to my friends because they probably won't get upset, so I just go to my friends instead of my family

Relying on friends for support, however, was not unproblematic for Lauren. She later remarks

> most of my friends were more concerned with Twitter and other forms of social media than family, and that only one of my friends – who had a disabled grandfather – could "relate" to me

* All names have been changed to preserve anonymity.

---

regard to the areas of unmet needs, in particular providing information, emotional support and normalisation of negative feelings. We feel that this commentary from a young family 'carer' serves as an example of how family members (who aren't designated carers as such) are still very much affected by a relative's progressive illness, don't necessarily have any support and may be invisible to services and other institutions, such as school.

Thinking Box

How might Lauren be affected by this situation?

How could Lauren be recognised as a tertiary care?

Why might Lauren be reluctant to discuss her grandmother's condition?

How might Laurens' situation affect school/college work?

In what ways can a nurse support Lauren?

It is important to think about 'lost opportunities' that we acknowledge; relationships with nurses and caregivers tend to evolve over time enhanced by continuity of care and communication methods. Many carers don't recognise themselves as being a 'carer', and as a consequence miss out on the support available. Those more likely to fall into this category are family caregivers who support people with mental health issues, children and young people, carers who are black and from other ethnic groups and those residing in more rural communities (Hare 2004). Of course, carers can be vulnerable and the possibilities for nurses to 'reach out' become even more challenging. Raising awareness and identifying primary carers has been an accepted endeavour, with carer leads and care champions located in GP practices (Greenwood et al. 2010). At the same time, some acute NHS Trusts have partnered with local carer centres that offer carer awareness training for all staff. This, in our view is good practice and highlights what is possible. In Scotland, Jarvis and McIntosh (2015), a district nurse and carer support worker, have set up a pilot care clinic to assess carers' own health and information needs. Their evaluation has shown that emotional support can make a difference alongside the culture of carer awareness and that carers' health checks promote well-being. Potential exists in undertaking carer health checks to explore ways to help carers re-construct their own identity and concerns about 'loss of self'.

As we discussed in Chapter 6, opportunities exist in attending support groups, writing blogs and journals and connecting through social media in attaining one's identity (partial for many carers) and reclaiming a sense of self. Use of telehealth may be helpful in determining the type of relationships – whether distant or close – between carers and nurses. In addition, more home-based care and changes in life expectancy technology can play a crucial role in supporting caregivers. Interestingly, North American and Scandinavian countries are the leading countries in offering telecare and technology to patients and family carers. A recent study undertaken in Norway by Solli et al. (2015) on the relationship between nurse and caregivers through telecare found that as a communication medium telecare helped bridge the support gap and the partnership roles evolved over time. What is interesting is that there was a notable shift in the power differential in that mutual respect unfolded with carers and nurses learning from one another. Telecare is a computer-mediated communication with web forums and web cameras; the carers were those caring for loved ones with dementia or strokes. The service was flexible and offered relationships that could become close or distant depending on the carer's attitude towards telecare as a service. The support offered demonstrated usefulness in terms of carer's physical and emotional problems. Again, one cannot assume from a generational cultural perspective whether telecare or technology is appealing or not. Consideration of the suitability of any communication or support method requires dialogue with a caregiver, and over time their preference may change. In part, this may reflect the nature of the carer's role and tasks, which inevitability are highly connected to the illness trajectory and illness-related challenges.

Rolland (1987) offers a useful illness typology model in terms of linking biological and psychosocial demands of chronic illness upon patients and their family; the illness patterns can vary in relation to onset, course, outcome, incapacitation and the level of uncertainty. Within this illness trajectory or patterns, there are three major time phases of illness – crisis, chronic and terminal. In each phase, meanings and implications have profound effects on families and it is in this context that Rolland and Wash (2006) suggest that illness does not get in the way of normality and family life. Importantly, they suggest that one attempts to 'keep the illness in its place' in that a balance is struck between being self and the limitations brought by the illness. Of course, this can be a challenge or problem depending on your mindset, and many other factors come into play in terms of family function (Chapter 2) and responses (Chapters 3 through 5), but increased support and understanding by nurses can really make a difference. Supporting families and carers cannot be underestimated for its reach and worth as when it happens it makes a huge difference to people's lives. However, the manner in which nurses interact and approach families and carers matters; kindness and thoughtfulness go a long way. We urge you to grasp opportunities, for we believe there are plenty, indeed more than what is covered in this chapter.

Finally, we would like to end this book with a short poem written by a group of student nurses in response to our teaching sessions on raising awareness of carers.

The Silent Carer

Hello I'm Sarah and I'm just seven
I don't want my mum to go to heaven
At home I always try my best
But at school it seems I always fail my tests
My teacher sees me as 'just a bad kid'
If only she knew what I really did!
My friends play out and have a good time
But I can never invite them to mine
I cook, clean and wash my mum
Then go to bed when I'm done
I don't whinge or moan I just pray
That they don't take my mum away
As a nurse we can make a difference
To reduce her commitments
To make her life so much fairer
We need to raise the awareness of the *Silent Carer*!

Key Points

- Opportunities exist to improve recognition and the value of caregivers involvement in the care of their loved ones – patients.
- A triad partnership comprising the patient, nurse and caregiver (family) strengthens relationships and experiences for all.
- Opportunities such as visitation strategies and protected mealtimes could benefit from research and evaluations that take into account close family and caregivers roles and needs alongside those of patients.
- Discharge planning requires early communication with families and carers in order to facilitate effective and safe transfer of care.
- Attributes such as kindness, thoughtfulness and caring towards supporting families and carers are fundamental to nursing in working *with* carers and families.

Chapter Summary

As nurses, we spend a great deal of our time with patients, as we adopt therapeutic relationships in the 'being' of nursing. In so doing, we draw upon our 'human pull', and this this give us privilege to enter their lives. At the same time an integral aspect of 'being', but also the 'doing', of nursing is the engagement and inclusion of family and carers. With this in mind, throughout this chapter, we have tried to convey some examples of opportunities where by primarily nurses can make improvements. Emphasis has been placed upon triad partnerships and consideration of the triangle of care, because when this is applied, the impact is huge and far reaching. Many of the carers we have spoken to over the years repeatedly state 'we just wish to be seen, to be valued and included as we are here to help'. As Lowson et al. (2013) found, many carers move from 'conductor to second fiddle' in their movement between home and hospital and back again. We can all make some small but profound changes and we hope that this final chapter offers insights to be able to do just that.

References

Agard AS, Egerod I, Tonnesen E and Lomborg K. (2015) From spouse to caregiver and back: A grounded theory study of post-intensive care unit spousal caregiving. *Journal of Advanced Nursing* 71(8): 1892–1903.

Agard SA and Maindl HT. (2009) Interacting with relatives in intensive care unit. Nurses' perceptions of a challenging task. *Nursing in Critical Care* 14(4): 264–272.

Allen K. (2004) Recognising and managing adult patients who are critically sick. *Nursing Times* 100: 34–37.

BBC. (2011) BBC news item. http://www.bbc.co.uk/news/health-15052636 (accessed 14 July 2015).

Benner P, Hooper-Kyriakidis P and Stannard D. (1999) *Clinical Wisdom and Interventions in Critical Care.* Philadelphia, PA: WB Saunders.

Borthwick R, Newbronner L and Stuttard L. (2009) 'Out of Hospital': A scoping study of services for carers of people being discharged from hospital. *Health & Social Care in the Community* 17(4): 335–349.

Bradby M. (2014) Community nurses supporting carers: A new online resource from the Queen's Nursing Institute. *British Journal of Community Nursing* 19(3): 142–143.

Bube P. (2002) The role of the family in in-patient care: A mostly modest proposal. *The Internet Journal of Law, Healthcare and Ethics* 1(2).

Carers Trust. (2010) *The Triangle of Care: Carers Included: A Guide to Best Practice in Acute Mental Health Care.* London, UK: Carers Trust. http://www.rcn.org.uk/:data/assets/pdf_file/0009/549063/Triangle_of_Care_-_Carers_Included_Sept_2013.pdf (accessed 17 July 2015).

Dalton JM. (2003) Development and testing of the theory of collaborative decision-making in nursing practice for triads. *Journal of Advanced Nursing* 41(1): 22–33.

Department of Health. (2003) *Discharge from Hospital: Pathway, Process and Practice.* London, UK: Department of Health.

Department of Health. (2007) *Improving Nutrition Care: A Joint Action Plan from the Department of Health and the Nutrition Summit Stakeholders.* London, UK: Department of Health.

Department of Health. (2010) *Ready to Go: Planning the Discharge and the Transfer of Patients from Hospital and Intermediate Care.* Leeds, UK: Department of Health.

Department of Health. (2012) *Compassion in Practice: Nursing, Midwifery and Care Staff. Our Vision and Strategy.* London, UK: The Stationery Office.

Department of Health. (2013) *The NHS Friends and Family Test: Publication Guidance.* London, UK: The Stationery Office.

Dewar B and Christley Y. (2013) A critical analysis of compassion in practice. *Nursing Standard* 28(10): 46–50.

Francis R. (2013) Report of the Mid Staffordshire NHS Foundation Trust Public Inquiry. Present and Future, Vol. 3. London, UK: The Stationery Office. http://webarchive. nationalarchives.gov.uk/20150407084003/http://www.midstaffspublicinquiry.com/ report (accessed 17 July 2015).

Galvin E, Boyer L, Schwartz PK, Jones MW, Mooney P, Warwick J and Davis J. (2000) Challenging the precepts of family centered care: Testing a philosophy. *Pediatric Nursing* 26(6): 625–632.

Greenwood N, Mackenzie A, Habbi R, Atkins C and Jones R. (2010) General practitioners and carers: A questionnaire survey of attitudes, awareness of issues, barriers and enablers to provision of services. *BMC Family Practice* 11: 100.

Hare P. (2004) Keeping carers healthy: The role of community nurses and colleagues. *British Journal of Community Nursing* 9(4): 155–159.

Hickson M, Connolly A and Whelan K. (2011) Impact of protected mealtimes on ward mealtime environment, patient experience and nutrient intake in hospitalised patients. *Journal of Human* Nutrition and *Dietetics* 24: 370–374.

Jarvis J and McIntosh G. (2015) Carers' health clinic initiative in Edinburgh: Pilot evaluation. *British Journal of Community Nursing* 12(9): 416–421.

Keen D and Knox M. (2004) Approach to challenging behaviour: A family affair. *Journal of Intellectual and Developmental Disability* 29(1): 52–64.

Levine C. (2004) *Always on Call: When Illness Turns Families into Caregivers,* 2nd ed. Nashville, TN: Vanderbilt University Press.

Lowson E, Hanratty B, Holmes L, Addington-Hall J, Grande G, Payne S and Seymour J. (2013) From 'conductor' to 'second fiddle': Older adult care recipients' perspectives on transitions in family caring at hospital admission. *International Journal of Nursing Studies* 50(9): 1197–1205.

Mottram A. (2011) 'They are marvellous with you whilst you are in but the aftercare is rubbish': A grounded theory study of patients' and their carers' experiences after discharge following day surgery. *Journal of Clinical Nursing* 20: 3143–3151.

Nash L. (2002) The effects of visitors on a postnatal ward. *The Practising Midwife* 5: 20–21.

National Patient Safety Agency (NPSA). (2006) Protected mealtimes review: Findings and recommendations report. http://www.nrls.npsa.nhs.uk/resources/?entryid45=59806 (accessed 17 July 2015).

Reinhard SC, Given B, Huhtala Petlick N and Bemis A. (2008) Chapter 14: Supporting family caregivers in providing care. In: R. G. Huges (Ed.) *Patient Safety and Quality: An Evidence-Based Handbook for Nurses.* Rockville, MD: Agency for Healthcare Research and Quality.

Resuscitation Council (UK) and European Research Council. (2000) *ALS Manual.* London, UK: RCUK/ERC.

Rolland JS. (1987) Chronic illness and the life cycle: A conceptual framework. *Family Process* 26: 203–221.

Rolland JS and Wash F. (2006) Facilitating family resilience with childhood illness and disability. *Current Opinion in Pediatrics* 18: 527–538.

Slatyer S, Toye C, Popescu A, Young J, Matthews A, Hill A and Williamson DJ. (2013) Early re-presentation to hospital after discharge from an acute medical unit: Perspectives of older patients, their family caregivers and health professionals. *Journal of Clinical Nursing* 22: 445–455.

Solli H, Hvalvik S, Torunn I and Helleso R. (2015) Characteristics of the relationship that develops from nurse-caregiver communication during telecare. *Journal of Clinical Nursing* 24(13–14): 1995–2004.

Stone K. (2014) Enhancing preparedness and satisfaction of caregivers of patients discharged from an inpatient rehabilitation facility using an interactive website. *Rehabilitation Nursing* 39: 76–85.

Stratton RJ et al. (2003) *Disease-Related Malnutrition: An Evidence-Based Approach to Treatment.* Wallingford, UK: CABI Publishing.

The Kings Fund. (2013) *Patient-Centred Leadership: Rediscovering Our Purpose.* London, UK: The Kings Fund.

Tobiano G, Chaboyer W and McMurray A. (2012) Family members' perceptions of the nursing bedside handover. *Journal of Clinical Nursing* 22: 192–200.

Turnbull AP and Turnbull HR. (2001) *Families, Professionals, and Exceptionality: Collaborating for Empowerment*, 4th ed. Upper Saddle River, NJ: Merrill/Prentice-Hall.

UK Government. (2008) Carers at the heart of 21st-century families and communities. http://tinyurl.com/qaf2m8p (accessed 24 February 2014).

Walker E and Dewar BJ. (2001) How do we facilitate carers' involvement in decision making? *Journal of Advanced Nursing* 34(3): 329–337.

Wray J. (2011) Bouncing back? An ethnographic study exploring the context of care and recovery after birth through the experiences and voices of mothers, Unpublished PhD thesis. Salford, UK: The University of Salford.

Wray J. (2012) Impact of place upon celebration of birth – Experiences of new mothers on a postnatal ward. *MIDIRS Midwifery Digest* 23(3): 357–361.

Useful Links

The **Queen's Nursing Institute** has developed three free online resources to support nurses who work with carers: http://www.qni.org.uk/supporting_carers.

Salford Carers Centre has a team of specialist support workers who will contact the carers to offer practical or emotional support. The centre has developed a Carers Links programme to embed 'carer awareness' within teams. All local GP surgeries have a Carers Link worker and plans are to extend this network to pharmacies and a local NHS hospital and NHS community service: www.salfordcarerscentre.co.uk.

Index